HAPPY MAMA POSTPARTUM SELF-CARE

NAVIGATING THE FIRST 12 WEEKS TO RECHARGE,
REFRESH, AND NURTURE FOR A SMOOTH
TRANSITION TO HEALTHY MOTHERHOOD

ROBYN WELLER, MSN, CNM

CONTENTS

DISCLAIMER

This book is inclusive for everyone. I know that not all birthing humans identify as moms. And that not all moms have birthed humans. However, I use the term "mom" for simplicity. I acknowledge my biases.

I may use words like breastfeeding instead of chest-feeding, again for simplicity, but know that I am supportive of all humans in the birth and new baby world. Inclusivity is key and the self-care advice in this book applies to anyone and everyone who needs it.

INTRODUCTION

There is nothing like bringing a new baby into the world. You spend years imagining it and months preparing for it. You have a nursery. You have a crib. You have cute clothes folded into a dresser and stacks of diapers ready to go. You learned how to breathe through the pain and what contractions feel like. Maybe you felt contractions, thought you were in labor, then got sent home to wait for the real thing! But once you give birth and hold that baby in your arms, you feel something you have never felt before.

Pure, unbridled fear.

Okay, I am kidding! Partially. Everyone talks about how much love they feel when holding their baby, which is great! But not everyone feels that way. Some moms have traumatic births and cannot even see their babies immediately. Some cradle them and do not feel that bond because they need to let it develop over time. Some feel love but are overwhelmed by not knowing what to do next. You can prepare for a baby as long as you want, for months or years. However, once you actually have a baby, things get real!

When I brought my first baby home, I remember walking through the door and gently placing the carrier on the kitchen table. I remember looking at her, still strapped in, and thinking, *now what? What should I do?* I was supposed to know what I was doing because of my profession, but I was also clueless. This gorgeous sweet little creature was sleeping like a potato, and I had no idea what to consider doing next. When you are there in that moment, real life is wildly different from what you read in baby books, saw online, and even envisioned for yourself.

Most pregnancy books talk about the preparation stages. Maybe the birth. But women need to be honest about what comes next. I love the saying, "The days are long, the nights an eternity, and the years go by in a blink." I have found this phrase is no joke—sometimes you may feel you cannot take one more breath because you are so tired, yet you know you need to push on for your baby. However, even that may not feel like enough when running on empty.

There is no need to sugarcoat motherhood and make it seem like the best time in your life. If that is what it is for you, that's great! But not everyone has that experience, and being honest about all the possibilities can make the difference between a new mother accepting herself and rolling with the punches or feeling beat down like she will never be a good parent. Honesty does not have to be harsh; it just needs to be a chance to let mothers feel what they are going through and understand that they are okay and that everything will be okay.

The reality of new motherhood is that everything changes. You might feel like an entirely different person, which can be good. After all, your focus is now on your newborn and giving them the best life possible. However, there are other changes that are not so good, like changes to your body. Some women legitimately bounce back to their non-pregnant selves. Some book gym time or hire trainers. Some do everything anyone has ever thought of or told them to do and still find that their body has changed shape and feels foreign. Your hair texture can change. Your tastes can change! Maybe you used to love pineapple, and now it makes you sick. It is weird, but that is what pregnancy, hormones, and a significant life change can do to you.

The first 12 weeks after giving birth is called the fourth trimester, and the fact that it has a legitimate name should help you realize how serious it is. This period is just as important as the first three trimesters when you were nurturing your baby inside you. Now you have to parent a newborn while still taking care of yourself. Unfortunately, many healthcare entities feel like pregnancy care ends once you give birth and allow the follow-up appointments for the mother to slack off. Mothers rarely prioritize themselves at this point, too, since they are worried about breastfeeding, is the baby gaining weight, how many wet diapers were there, is the baby pooping enough, is the baby pooping too much, is that what the umbilical cord is supposed to look like, and everything else that they can imagine worrying about. All this stems from the desire to do whatever it takes to get their baby on the right track for growth.

It is easy to let things go when you feel overwhelmed with keeping things together at home for your baby and getting to their appointments. Trying to get yourself to a postpartum follow-up appointment seems like something you can easily take off your plate to give yourself less stress and more time to be with your baby. However, this visit is crucial because your provider can check your body to ensure you are healing correctly. They can ask questions about your mindset and emotional stability. They can provide insight into your feelings to understand if it is normal, if it will pass, if you need professional help or more family support—or all of the above!

Ideally, postpartum care would be an ongoing process. However, there is typically just one follow-up visit at six weeks. Six weeks is a month and a half, and when you are learning how to parent a newborn, every minute can feel like an hour. Waiting this long for professional assistance is not the best option. Regular support and medical attention within a week or two after birth can significantly improve your transition to motherhood. Another appointment in the next three or four months gives you time to adjust to your new life, adapt to your baby, and see what issues you might need more help with. This also gives you time to settle into your new body and understand what changes you are facing regarding your physical health.

During the first 12 weeks of motherhood, you need to focus on specific realms of your life, including

- physical recovery
- newborn care
- sleep and fatigue
- mental health
- diet and exercise
- family planning

You can read about many of these issues in various parenting books, but they often make you feel guilty for the way you might not accept all those sterile answers. Let's also address, beyond just books, the endless void of social media. Can we all collectively lower the bar, not strive to look like we just got out of the salon?

You know what I would like to see?

Real photos. I want to see a picture of a real mama in her adult diapers, with circles under her eyes for days, trying to figure out how the damn breast pump works!

I will be honest: The truth is that motherhood is hard and gritty, and while it is a rewarding experience for most mothers, the process is not that straightforward. This book will help you understand how you can prioritize your fourth trimester to be the time you need to heal physically and emotionally, with honest advice from moms who have had dramatically different experiences with newborns.

One important thing to remember is that every experience is different. I will cover as much as possible here, and just from these examples, you will see how drastically each mother's experience can vary. You might see yourself in some of these stories. You might realize you do not have it as bad or feel like you have it worse. Regardless, I am here to help. And you should know that every birth is different, even yours. I have helped first-time moms with breezy deliveries who seem to bounce back immediately. Then I have seen first-time moms unable to follow their birth plan and struggle after that point. I have seen the same thing happen to mothers giving birth to their second and third children. Childbirth and postpartum, fortunately, or unfortunately, are not like riding a bike. You can have a fantastic delivery and be so excited for your second baby just to have a completely different experience. That is why it is crucial to remember that each birth is different, and sometimes you must roll with it. This book is the ultimate guide to helping you understand what you are going through now, so you will want to keep it on hand as you progress through pregnancy and the fourth trimester.

Why should you listen to me about any of this?

I am a Certified Nurse Midwife with over 20 years of experience in women's health. There are a few different types of midwives with different educational paths and formal titles. My path began with a bachelor's degree in nursing. I then worked in both hospital and clinic settings as a Registered Nurse.

After five years, I knew I was ready to pursue my true calling and begin my journey to become a Certified Nurse Midwife. I enrolled in a midwifery program in Kentucky at the Frontier School of Nursing and Case Western Reserve University in Ohio. I eventually graduated with a master's degree in nursing and a certificate in midwifery. This allowed me to sit for another super stressful and challenging national board exam (I passed!) and thus became a Certified Nurse Midwife.

People may recognize the term Nurse Practitioner more readily. Certified Nurse Midwives are like that but also specialize in pregnancy and birth. Although what we are allowed to do varies from state to state, we generally (and I specifically) are authorized to diagnose, write prescriptions, perform exams, and, obviously, deliver babies.

Professionally speaking, I have experience working in adolescent mental health facilities, family planning clinics, private practice hospitals, and large HMOs. I have worked at hospitals' labor and delivery units, postpartum units, and neonatal intensive care units (NICUs). Most of my career has been as a hospital-based midwife, working in a clinic setting and caring for women of all ages. Of course, I spend a lot of time helping mamas deliver, and at this point, I have "caught" over 2000 babies.

Okay, so in real life, what do I do now?

Do I do homebirths in swimming pools? Answer: I do not, but if that is how you want to deliver your baby, more power to you.

Am I super "crunchy" and only take care of non-medicated birthing humans? Answer: No. I deliver babies in a hospital. With and without medication, that is up to you, and I support both choices.

Do I only deliver babies? Answer: No. I perform the full suite of maternal care, including preconception, postpartum, and all the visits in between. I also take care of well-women visits, including paps, infections, birth control, and peri and post-menopause. Essentially if you have a uterus and vagina, I can care for you!

When describing myself to my patients, I consider myself "The midwife in the middle." I am a bit crunchy, but I also read papers in scientific journals and focus on evidence-based studies. When I hear off-the-wall stuff about some new idea that claims to improve your birthing experience, I like to say, "Interesting. Did you read about that in a peer-reviewed journal? Let's look into that!"

Who do I see as far as perinatal care? My fellow certified nurse midwife colleagues and I care for 80% of women in the middle. Typically, not the swimming pool in the living room, intervention free-birth crowd. If you had that, great! I support your choice. I personally work in a hospital. I also do not handle the super high-risk crowd either. The physicians get to handle those.

Perhaps most importantly, I have given birth to four babies of my own and lived through some difficult stuff.

I tell all mamas, especially the not-their-first-birth mamas-to-be, that every birth is different. That has certainly been the case for me! I have had long, induced, "epiduralized" births. I have also had a non-medicated, no time for drugs, fast and furious birth. I have battled debilitating postpartum depression and anxiety. I have experienced early pregnancy vomiting until I needed IVs, gestational diabetes, working ridiculous hours with maternity belts on, painful nipples, mastitis, angry hemorrhoids, gallons of my own tears, and so many sleeping nights—fatigue with a capital F.

I wrote this book because I have been there, done that, and understand how frightening and overwhelming it can feel. I take the perspective of both a mom and a clinician. I have seen the good and the bad and occasionally the ugly. I came out on the other side myself and have helped others get there too. Mainly I wrote this book to help you navigate whatever you are going through.

In this book, you will get honest advice from professionals and tips and tricks from moms who have been there and done that. While reading some of the classic pregnancy books is a great way to get a solid foundation of knowledge before you give birth, you want something real when navigating those late-night feedings after hardly getting enough sleep to function. You need a book that tells it like it is, like friends cheering you on from the pages. This book is exactly what you need. Let's get real about motherhood and raising a newborn while prioritizing your physical and emotional health during the fourth trimester. Wherever you are in your journey of transitioning to motherhood, rest assured that it is just the right spot for you. Just where you are supposed to be. And you are not alone, so let's do this together.

Certainly, great pregnancy and parenting sites, books, blogs, and podcasts are available for reality and encouragement. Still, it is hard to sift through the junk and find the good stuff —especially when you already feel so strapped for time as a new mother. This book is the real deal: no fluff and buff. You can bounce around from chapter to chapter. Put stickies in spots you want your partner to read or hear. Highlight phrases that stick out to you and help you feel like a person instead of a baby servant. Come back to the same section over and over if it is something you need to remind yourself. There is no wrong way to read this book, so jump in and see what makes the most impact.

1

THRIVING IN MOTHERHOOD— WHY POSTPARTUM SELF-CARE MATTERS

Taking care of yourself doesn't mean me first; it means me too.

— L.R. KNOST

D id you know that carrying a baby is the equivalent of running a 40-week marathon? If you wonder why you felt so tired for so long, there is a good reason why. Duke University researchers collected data from Race Across the USA, a 120-day, 3000-mile race that covers approximately a marathon a day for six days per week. They investigated metabolic rates for participants in the event. For context, the highest BMR a human can sustain is 2.5, meaning the average adult burns 4,000 calories daily. They compared it to pregnant mothers who typically experience a 2.2 BMR (The Healthy Mommy, 2019). Pregnant women are operating nearly at the max BMR for nine months, which definitely sounds like a workout. You do not need me to tell you how exhausting pregnancy is, but sometimes it helps to have comparisons like this to know you are not imagining things—it is truly a difficult time in your life. And then you have to give birth, and then you have to care for a newborn, and then you have to raise a child... Well, let's not get ahead of ourselves.

Mothers often feel like they are being selfish when they care for themselves. After all, you have a newborn to care for now —shouldn't that be your focus? Well, yes and no. You need to care for your baby but cannot help anyone if you are completely depleted. We have all heard the saying, "Put your oxygen mask on first before helping others." I want to ingrain this in your mind. If Mama is doing poorly, the family unit will most likely follow suit.

I tell pregnant people worrying too much about nutrition that the baby will get what they need in utero. They take from you to grow, so you do not need to worry about them —ensure you are getting what you need. The same holds true once the baby is born. You will feed them, cuddle them, change them, burp them, love them—yes, yes, of course! However, you must also feed yourself, put yourself to bed, support yourself, and love yourself. That is why postpartum self-care matters.

PREGNANCY AND POSTPARTUM CARE IN THE UNITED STATES

Before we get to the meat of the book, I feel I should issue a disclaimer: Healthcare in the United States sucks. Especially for pregnant people. And postpartum care? Forget it! Finding quality postpartum care can feel like seeing a unicorn leap across the sky!

Millions of women give birth annually in the United States, and most experience healthy pregnancies and childbirth. However, despite its reputation as a developed country, there are an increasing number of complications during people's pregnancies and birth experiences (BlueCross BlueShield, 2020).

A study from BlueCross BlueShield pulled statistics from 1.8 million pregnancies between 2014 to 2018. The women were aged 18 to 44 and had commercial insurance. The study found that birth complications did not increase with age, so the statistics applied to the entire pool. The study found that the number of women experiencing both pregnancy and childbirth complications increased by 31.5%, and the number of women diagnosed with postpartum depression increased by 30% (BlueCross BlueShield, 2020).

Sadly, the mortality rate for women during childbirth in the United States is increasing. It is multifactor in reasons, but the numbers are bleak. In 2021, there were 32.9 deaths for every 100,000 live births, up from 23.8 in 2020 and 20.1 in 2019. That statistic more than doubles to 69.9 for Black women. This statistic does increase with age, at 20.4 deaths per 100,000 live births for mothers younger than 25, 31.3 for those 25 to 39, and 138.5 for anyone over 40 (Hoyert, 2023).

The United States has the highest maternal death rate of any developed country. Our numbers are staying stable or rising compared to other countries that are taking action to make those death rates decline (The Commonwealth Fund, 2020). The causes of these deaths include but are not limited to:

- inadequate prenatal care
- high rate of cesarean sections
- probability of chronic illness
- missed opportunities for treatment
- systemic racism

About 14% of women did not receive prenatal care in their first trimester because of a lack of appointment availability, nearby providers, or no way to get to the appointment. For those reasons, almost one-third of the respondents said they attended less than the ten recommended prenatal visits. Of those groups, a quarter went on to experience childbirth complications (BlueCross BlueShield, 2020).

After giving birth, 4% of women said they did not receive any postpartum care, and 26% said they were not screened for postpartum depression (BlueCross BlueShield, 2020). 6.9 million women have little to no access to maternal healthcare. Compared to other developed countries, the overall maternal and infant healthcare system in the United States gets a grade of C-, which is far from decent (March of Dimes, n.d.).

Other countries begin empowering pregnant people for parenthood at 22 or 34 weeks, with countries like Finland offering an impressive box of newborn essentials and Spain offering a mother's passport, including monthly check-ins with a midwife. Many countries encourage at least 30 days of complete rest for new mothers, which can decrease the odds of experiencing postpartum depression (Major, 2020).

Think of other medical situations in the United States. Someone who goes in for knee surgery may stay several nights in the hospital, then have up to six weeks of rest at home with physical therapy visits. New mothers rarely get this type of treatment, and if they do get a more extended hospital stay and recovery time, it is often something they have to fight for and explain to others. Societal pressures make new moms feel like they must immediately bounce back, physically and emotionally, and start "doing it all" to prove or validate their worth.

Part of the problem here is the need for paid maternity leave in the United States. Only 14% of employees get paid leave, and 40% do not qualify for the Family Medical Leave Act (FMLA). Considering these facts, it is unsurprising that one out of four new mothers return to work ten days after having their baby (Major, 2020).

I was a labor and delivery nurse in Montana when I had my second child. I had to go back to work between four and five weeks postpartum. My midwife wanted me to stay out longer, but I could not afford it, even with a good job. I needed a roof over our heads, food in the fridge, and to pay for childcare. Montana does not have pregnancy disability, so if you did not have enough vacation time, you had to deal with a complete loss of income or go back to work. If I did want to use the 12 weeks of FMLA, in addition to not getting paid, I would have had to pay my employer for my healthcare benefits during my time off.

The point of this section is to provide a foundation for the book. You may or may not have access to a stellar provider who gives you thorough checkups and talks you through the fourth trimester. You may be doing this all on your own, so I am trying to serve as a source of knowledge based on more than 20 years of experience as a midwife, plus my decades of research.

With this information in mind, I will start slowly with some background information about the fourth trimester, including things you may experience and how you can be proactive in caring for yourself after childbirth.

THE IMPORTANCE OF EARLY POSTPARTUM SELF-CARE INTERVENTIONS

The key to making it through this period without losing it centers on self-care. Many mothers overlook themselves as they focus on caring for others, but you need to take it slow and be gracious with yourself. This section will briefly touch on some of the more important aspects of self-care, but this is to touch on the point that it is so needed. Additional chapters will go over each aspect in more detail.

The immediate postpartum period lasts about six to eight weeks, starting after you give birth and ending when your body has mostly healed, and you are fully functioning. This process involves many mental, emotional, and physical changes. You have to rebuild your physical and mental strength. It would be best to focus on resting, getting plenty of nutrition, and relying on your support system to empower you to heal fully. However, this is the start of your postpartum journey, not the end!

Rest

Everyone knows that new parents need rest, just as everyone also knows that they rarely get it! Your baby does not pay attention to the clock or consider your needs independently. They wake up every three hours or so, wanting food, a clean diaper, and a cuddle. You might feel like you are trying to appease a tiny dictator who cannot calmly tell you what they need right there and then. Their main form of communication early on is crying, which can initially feel overwhelming, especially if it is your first baby. You cannot get a whole night of sleep if you are awake every three hours, caring for your little one.

We will talk about rest a lot in this book because it is so crucial for new mamas. It may seem repetitive, but it is because it is so important, and we want to ensure you understand why.

Instead of expecting to get eight hours of sleep to feel human, it is best to adjust your expectations from the start. "Sleep when the baby sleeps" is advice you will hear from everyone, whether they are a parent, grandparent, doctor, midwife, or random person on the street—everyone knows that phrase because it is true. The only chance you have to sleep is when the baby is asleep. Otherwise, you are caring for them.

As someone who has worked night shifts for most of my career, before the birth of my first child, I thought the talk of "fatigue" from caring for a baby was cute but silly. I had been "fatigued" at 3:45 AM, nine hours into a shift that would not end for another three hours. Yea, I was tired, and so was everyone else. We all just pushed through it. I had no idea the level of pure unadulterated fatigue that I would be experiencing as a new parent. Sure, I could pull off work with little sleep, but I eventually had time to catch up. I also did not have a large pancake size wound in my uterus that was trying to heal, sutures in my vagina, and the stress of making enough breast milk to sustain another human.

The best "hack" for getting through those sleepless nights and the tidal wave of fatigue is the support of a partner, family, or friends. If possible, you should only focus on feeding the baby and resting. Remember, you just went through pregnancy and childbirth. Sure, other people support you in various ways, but their bodies are not trying to adapt to the change and heal after delivery, so they are capable of more than you. Resting is vital for your body's healing, so you do not need to be afraid to ask for help. If you have people with you in the hospital, perhaps eager grandparents, gently encourage them to go home and rest up. It is like changing shifts, with you giving birth while your support team sleeps, then they can come on board and take over so you can rest and start recovery. Other people can change diapers, and everyone loves to cuddle a newborn. You will get quality time with your baby when you feed them, and then you can rest up to become your best self.

While much of this advice is geared toward first-time moms, you should consider how it can impact you, even if this is not your first baby. I felt like I got less and less support with each child I had (I have four). Maybe it was because people thought I knew what I was doing. However, just because I could change a diaper in my sleep blindfolded with my hands tied behind my back did not mean that I was not healing and still needed rest and care. It is like how people do not tend to throw baby showers for second, third, and fourth babies because they assume you have everything you need. But it can be more work with the second (or more) child because you now have older kids to manage along with your newborn.

As a provider, if I could write a "prescription" for sleep, I would. Uninterrupted sleep. If people saw that taped to your fridge on an official script pad, they would take it more seriously. There is no underestimating the power of quality rest.

Let me pause here and clarify- it is hard to sleep when the baby sleeps. You might not be tired at that point, or more accurately, you are probably so overly tired that you feel hyped up again. You may want to make a batch of meals to freeze or deep clean the kitchen like you have been putting off. My advice? Do not. Seriously. You might want to keep your home intact all around you, but it is not worth it at this moment. If there is ever a time in your life when you deserve (and get!) a pass on domestic responsibilities, this is it! And the change needs to start with us. Leave a sink of dirty dishes as your way of making a stand for new moms and feel good about it! There will be plenty of time to clean or just a thought, let your partner clean! However, now is not that time because you need to rest. Before you know it, the baby will be awake again and needing you, so take advantage of every moment. Even if you do not sleep, just rest! Once you let other things go, you might find that you are a master of getting 10 minutes of sleep at a time and using that rest as fuel to make it to the next naptime.

Looking back, this is one of my biggest regrets. I should have had conversations with my support team before I was so behind the eight ball that my eyeballs would not stay open. I should have "allocated" more jobs to my support people. I should have been much more specific with my partner on what needs were not being met so that I could sleep and rest more, not just for myself, but so I could be the best for all of us.

Another way to maximize your sleep is to keep the baby near your bed. When they wake up to eat, you can feed them without getting up and walking to another room. The American Academy of Pediatrics recently updated its safe sleep recommendations. They do not recommend having the baby sleep in your bed but do recommend that you keep the baby's crib in your room for the first six months (American Academy of Pediatrics, 2022). If you have room, put that kid right next to your bed so you do not have to get out to pick them up.

Another hack to maximizing potential rest time is to take advantage of guests. New mothers commonly feel like they need to be the good host, sitting up with guests who want to see the new baby when they want to be alone, preferably sleeping. I know mothers who cannot stand to have someone visit their house without offering them a beverage and a snack. While these hostess skills are awe-inspiring, they are also exhausting. Depending on how much you trust your guests and if your partner is around, consider politely excusing yourself for a nap while you have company. I promise that if they are real friends who genuinely care about you, they will support your choice here.

I always tell patients that the only visitors they should have over the first few weeks after giving birth are people you can be topless around—that is the ultimate sign of trust! They are your people, and you can trust them with your baby. You will not feel pressure to clean the house and prepare snacks for them because they have already been with you through so much that there is no need to play hostess—they can handle you when you are being genuine. If you cannot ask someone to hand you an ice pack to put on your crotch, they can wait to meet your baby until you have recovered.

Since your new sleep schedule will throw off your circadian rhythm, it is best to get outside for at least a few minutes a day. Sun exposure will give your body vitamin D and help you naturally note the times of day to stay on track. You can bring your baby to get some vitamin D and fresh air. Ensure you keep them out of the direct sun; 15 minutes is standard, but you can talk to your provider about sunscreen and cover options to protect your baby outside (Terreri, 2018). However, going outside with your baby can boost your moods and energy levels while providing bonding time.

Nutrition

Rest gives your body enough opportunity to recover from pregnancy and childbirth, and when you pair rest with good nutrition, you will feel much better very quickly. Eating a balanced diet gives you plenty of energy and nutrition for yourself and your baby, especially if you are breastfeeding.

You should listen to your body and eat when you feel hungry, regardless of the concept of three-square meals or not eating in the middle of the night. After all, you are awake around the clock with your newborn, so what is time? Satisfy your body when hungry, and you will feel more empowered to parent. With such a random schedule, you might forget to make food at stereotypical mealtimes anyway, or you might get lucky and sleep through them, so eating when you are hungry is the best way to ensure you eat well.

Do not think about losing your pregnancy weight at this point. Your body can use the weight you gained during pregnancy to help recovery. Rapidly losing weight can actually harm you and your baby if you breastfeed because you will not have the nutrition necessary to support yourselves. Instead of trying to lose weight, focus on eating healthy foods, cutting out high-fat snacks, and getting a little appropriate exercise daily.

I tried to do a "clean eating challenge" when I had my last baby before returning to work. I "followed the plan," and my milk supply plummeted. Before having my baby, I had participated in multiple triathlons and long-distance endurance events and unrealistically felt ready to return to that physique. I was not secure in my mom bod, and I wanted to fit into clothing I did not need to fit into yet. I did not love the numbers on the scale. I felt all the typical unrealistic "pressure and expectations" that society places on new moms. My mindset was all wrong. I should have focused on all the healthy food I could have enjoyed instead of what I "should not have." Carbs are not evil, and there is such a thing as good fat! Plus, calorie-dense food can be healthy!

Exercise can help you reach your ideal weight more safely by staying active to boost your energy levels while ensuring you eat healthy foods. You can talk to your provider about what exercises are safe for you at certain stages in recovery, but light exercise is usually good for most new mothers. Slow and steady wins the race! You can walk around the neighborhood with your baby in a stroller. You can even walk laps in your backyard if you have the space. If you like a more structured exercise plan, check with your provider to see if you can do yoga at home while the baby naps or attend fitness classes at the gym. Many gyms offer classes for new mothers and childcare so you can attend (DiMaggio, n.d.). Remember, it took you 9 or 10 months to gain this weight. Plan on it taking at least that long to lose it. Slow and steady wins the race!

Along with the right foods, you need to stay hydrated post-partum, especially if you are breastfeeding. Some parents get incredibly thirsty while they nurse their babies like they are sucking them dry. Keep fresh water nearby so you can grab a big drink when you need one. I do not know about you, but I have seventy million water bottles at my house. If you do, too, ask someone to fill them up and spread them throughout the house. One next to the couch, the bed, the dining table, the bathroom, all over! And if plain water is not your jam (I think it tastes gross!), create some "spa water." Cut up some cucumber and add mint leaves or bits of fruit to liven it up so you have delicious water you are eager to drink, helping you stay hydrated. You can also drink milk to stay hydrated. If you get hungry when breastfeeding, keep snacks with water to keep your energy up during this slow time.

Support

I touched on this in the rest section because support is crucial for new mothers to have a chance to sleep. However, you can also welcome support in other ways. Right now, your primary focus should be your newborn and your recovery. Forget about making meals for everyone or keeping the house clean. Your partner can step up and do those tasks. If you are going at it alone, do not hesitate to ask a close friend or extended family member if they mind helping with specific duties. So many people want to help new mothers but must figure out what to offer without getting in the way. If you ask, the worst they can say is no!

When people ask if you need anything—and they will—tell them yes! However, give them specific ideas or tasks that you need. "Can you grab a rotisserie chicken from Costco and leave it at the door? We had a rough night last night." Or "Can you grab a pack of wipes and leave it at the door? We just need today to rest a bit extra." See what I did there? They can leave it at the door and give you time and space to recover.

Always communicate your needs with your helpers, whether they are friends and family or hired help. Let them know the main tasks you need them to do and ensure they will not get hurt feelings if you have to ask them for some space when you are having a rough day with the baby. If you prefer to avoid having other people in your home, consider getting help with tasks like shopping trips or yard work. And if you want to avoid meals and groceries, hello, food delivery! Uber, DoorDash, and Instacart can be lifesavers! They are also stellar gift ideas if people ask if there is anything they could do to help.

THE ROLE OF SOCIAL SUPPORT NETWORKS IN PROMOTING MATERNAL MENTAL HEALTH

Feeling like you are alone as you navigate new motherhood can feel bleak. Statistically, mothers with social support experience less stress (Henton & Swanson, 2023). They can turn to others when they need to vent or have someone watch the baby while they shower or rest. Having a support system also makes it more likely that women will not experience postpartum depression. Feeling overwhelmed by your new baby with no relief or breaks can send you toward depression or anxiety. Talking with other mothers is a great form of social support because they understand what you are going through. Talking with other *honest* mothers, who will not give you the fluffed up, I am trying to impress you version of things, is even better because there will be no holds barred in how they share the truth with you.

Isolation and loneliness have been shown to increase your risks for perinatal and postpartum depression (Billie Taylor, 2021). One of my dearest friends in Montana got me through some of the loneliest, darkest times as a fresh and depressed mom. She would show up at my house, pick things up, and mindlessly start cleaning. She would have me and the kids over for lunch, dinner, and playdates and let me sleep at her house. I will always be so grateful for her and the friendship that we still have!

Now I am sorry here but social media posts from influencer mothers are not a form of support. Those posts can be more damaging than you realize (Baker & Yang, 2018). While you can find practical support on parenting message boards, social media is another monster entirely (Jiang & Zhu, 2022). Many accounts want to put their best foot forward and promote envy, which is different from the mindset you need right now. If the post is from a trusted friend, who is also a new mom, and she is sharing how things are so hard, that is one thing. However, if the post is from somebody you do not know, with a bajillion followers, they are wearing makeup and look amazing... I am not sure that is serving you well at this moment in your life! You do not need to focus on anyone else, and you 100% do not need to impress anyone. Just get support for what you are dealing with.

New mothers can receive emotional support from their social support networks, which include spouses, family members, friends, and other mothers. People offering empathy, sympathy, and a listening ear can help ease feelings of loneliness, anxiety, and sadness. Having someone to discuss your thoughts and experiences is helpful to maternal mental health. It has also been shown that fears of being judged to be inadequate mothers can make it even more difficult for women to make authentic connections with others or to express negative feelings, increasing isolation and potential depression (Billie Taylor, 2021). You need your tribe! And they do exist. You may already have your "group," but if not, it is okay to start finding those friends. I know it can feel hard to make "new mom friends," but they are out there and ready to be your friend too!

Practical aid from social support networks, in addition to emotional support, can be incredibly helpful too. Helping with domestic duties, preparing food, or caring for the infant helps alleviate some of the stress and anxiety new mothers feel. This assistance enables you to concentrate on self-care and healing, lowering the chance of developing mental health difficulties.

New mothers can also benefit from social support networks in terms of knowledge and guidance. Access to correct and relevant information can boost a mother's confidence and minimize emotions of doubt and worry, whether it is sharing knowledge about newborn care, breastfeeding, or coping strategies for sleep deprivation.

Mothers can connect with others going through similar experiences by joining a social support network. Sharing tales, struggles, and triumphs can help normalize the spectrum of feelings and problems with parenthood. By lowering self-doubt and encouraging a sense of belonging, feeling understood and validated can lead to improved mental health.

Participating in peer support groups like new mothers' or postpartum support groups can have more advantages. These groups provide an organized atmosphere for women to discuss their experiences, learn from others, and receive support from others experiencing similar difficulties. Peer support groups can assist in alleviating feelings of isolation and foster a sense of belonging. Sometimes it also helps to have something on your calendar, breaking up the seemingly-endless stretch of feeding the baby, diapering the baby, and trying to sleep.

When it comes to forming a new social support group, I always encourage patients to give it a try! Go to that new mom stroller walk, babywearing group, meetup playdate. People show up to those expecting to meet new friends. It can be scary and overwhelming to consider getting out of your comfort zone, especially if you are an introvert. However, you can meet like-minded folks in the same boat as you! Another thing I like to mention is that by meeting parents who also just had a child, you will be meeting folks who may cross your path for a long time.

Your kids will likely be in school together. They may know of a daycare they love and has an opening. Having a child will create a new social circle in your life one way or another. Consider this a chance to get to know that group early. This can be a new friend group for you and very well could turn into friends for life.

Access to professional help, like healthcare providers, therapists, or counselors specializing in maternal mental health, can also come from social support networks. Hopefully, you love your provider and trust their recommendations, but hearing about other people's experiences is always lovely. They may recommend a pediatrician who aligns more with your values or know a therapist who makes them comfortable.

The social network is also vital because it may recognize signs of distress, encourage people to seek professional help and provide practical assistance by helping schedule appointments or caring for the newborn if you need to start some therapy.

UNDERSTANDING THE MOTHER WOUND

The Mother Wound is still a newer concept many have not heard of. However, it significantly affects how many people deal with postpartum and why self-care is so important. Donal Winnicott, a psychoanalyst, found that a mother's bond with her child is so strong that there is no infant alone, but always the infant and their mother (Lewis, 2020), meaning that the baby will always have a connection to their mother. It is a sweet concept, but there are many ramifications to this mindset. One is that the infant has the most substantial relationship with the mother, who is usually their primary caretaker. If the mother is not there emotionally for the children, they might experience the "mother wound." This can absolutely affect your experience with your postpartum time.

The mother wound is not a specific diagnosis but rather something you feel based on attachment theory. If you experience the mother wound in your childhood, you are more likely to have a similar relationship with your children. However, you can notice the signs and work to free yourself from the feelings to provide more for your offspring.

Some common feelings relating to the mother's wound include

- being unable to get comfort or security from your mother.
- feeling like you never had your mother's approval.
- acting nervous or scared around your mother.
- not getting emotional needs met by your mother.
- needing to take care of your mother emotionally or physically.

Any child can feel the mother wound, but daughters typically experience it differently, which they can then pass down to their children if it is left unresolved. The mother wound may exist if the mother cared for children physically without giving them love and security. The mother may not have given the children empathy or taught them how to manage their emotions. They may be critical of their children and expect the child to handle their needs independently. Mothers who experienced emotional or physical abuse, have untreated mental health conditions, or have an addiction may also pass the mother's wound on to their children.

Women who experience the mother wound may grow up with low self-esteem, a lack of emotional awareness, and an inability to soothe themselves. They may feel like they are not capable of being in a loving relationship. Growing up with secure attachment means you know how love feels and feel free to share it with others. You can feel your emotions, label them, and process them. You can calm yourself down without turning to others or needing drugs or alcohol to numb yourself. With a mother's relationship being one of the strongest in childhood, the lack of that relationship can mean that people do not feel confident enough to have deep, long-lasting relationships with others.

If you think you might have experienced the mother wound in childhood, there are ways you can find balance in your life as an adult and a new parent. One key is to allow yourself to feel emotions. Write about things you feel so you can take the time to understand what you feel and why before working through it. This will also help you develop self-awareness because you will feel more in touch with yourself and can cope with what you feel. Talking to a counselor or therapist can be an essential step. It can also help you to become a better parent as well. It is challenging to parent while you are still trying to heal from your childhood.

Above all, self-care is a significant part of healing from the mother wound. You are giving yourself the space to be your priority, even if your mother never gave you that grace. You take care of your needs and spend time getting in touch with yourself and your emotions.

MYTHS AND MISCONCEPTIONS ABOUT POSTPARTUM RECOVERY

There are so many myths and misconceptions about postpartum recovery. You might hear them from people you trust or think it is something you know, but it is always best to double-check the information to verify it is correct. Check out this list of common myths and see if you share any of these thoughts (Crouch, 2022).

- **You can drink too much water after delivery.** Many mothers think this, especially after a C-section. The myth says that less water can help your stitches heal faster. Cold water was thought to prevent the womb from shrinking to pre-pregnancy size, so new mothers were encouraged to consume warm drinks. However, there is no need to avoid a refreshing glass of cold water.
- **You should not eat ghee and milk after a C-section.** This myth seems the opposite of the breast milk myth, though there is some truth to it. You can eat ghee, milk, and dairy products, but too much can be unhealthy (Achwal, 2020).
- **You need to drink milk to produce breast milk.** This is a myth because you can drink plenty of water to make breast milk for your baby. However, drinking cow's milk or soy milk can increase your

milk supply and provide more nutrition than water alone, but you certainly do not have to.

- **You should not breastfeed when you are sick.** This is a myth because you will still provide the necessary nutrition for your baby even when you feel sick. Your illness will not pass through the breastmilk, so you can nurse or pump to feed your baby.

- **Speaking of all these breastfeeding myths, the biggest one is that it is easy.** People think that because most women can breastfeed, it is simple to do. That is not true. Some babies have trouble latching and getting enough milk. Some mothers do not produce enough milk. Sometimes it is too painful to breastfeed. While this method will give your baby great nutrition benefits, you do not need to beat yourself up about it or force it if things are not going smoothly.

- **Pain is normal in the postpartum stage.** This myth varies because you will experience some pain as your uterus shrinks, but overall, you should feel discomfort more than pain. Discomfort is a natural side effect of your body's healing. If you feel more intense pain, talk to your provider immediately.

- **The six-week checkup clears you to go back to normal.** Again, this myth has little truth because most providers clear mothers to exercise and have sex at this point. However, you most likely will not feel completely "normal" at this point. You were pregnant for around nine months, so expecting at least that long to recover is a good idea.

- **Your baby bump disappears after giving birth.** Huge myth, no pun intended! Your bump will decrease because you are not carrying your baby anymore. However, it can take six months to a year—or longer!—until you settle into your new mama bod. Maybe it will be the same as pre-pregnancy or something different, which is okay too!

- **You cannot get pregnant if you are breastfeeding.** While you most likely can have sex six weeks after giving birth, you will want to be just as careful about getting pregnant as at any other time. Your body makes prolactin to create milk, and that hormone can also stop you from ovulating and having a period, but it is not at all guaranteed. You can still get pregnant even if your period has not returned.

- **Everyone gets postpartum depression.** Many new parents feel the baby blues, but about 15% of mothers will experience postpartum depression. If you feel any of the symptoms written in the chapter reviewing postpartum depression (chapter 3), contact your provider for help and support.

- **Once you have a C-section, you can only give birth via C-section.** This was true in the past, but now it is safe for many women to have a vaginal birth after a cesarean (VBAC).

- **You cannot breastfeed after a C-section.** Since a C-section is a major surgery, the root of this myth is understandable. However, you can still find a comfortable way to breastfeed or pump after a C-section.
- **Spinal anesthesia can cause back pain in the future.** It is very rare for women to experience back pain for weeks or years after getting spinal anesthesia, so do not let that myth scare you off from creating your ideal birth plan.
- **C-sections lead to less bleeding and a lower chance of postpartum blues.** It would be nice if these myths were true since you have to undergo major surgery with a cesarean. However, you will still have vaginal bleeding after a C-section because the uterus lining sloughs off. Similarly, you have experienced a significant life change after giving birth, regardless of the method, so you can still experience postpartum mood issues and should stay aware of the possibilities.
- **Everyone's postpartum experience is the same.** In addition to having different experiences regarding the fourth trimester's moods and healing, women have drastically different backgrounds and cultures. The United States is a county of immigrants, and those people often bring their medical practices and beliefs to their childbirth experiences. For example, some cultures provide more family support for the

mother and infant. Some invite community elders to serve as birth attendants. In many countries, the new mother has three to five weeks of rest to ensure she heals with a lower risk of later injuries and illnesses (Dennis et al., 2007). Clearly, those differ from what many women in the United States experience, so it is understandable that they have many other cultural beliefs brought into the postpartum period.

HOW DOULAS CAN HELP

One thing I recommend to pregnant women is the help of a postpartum doula. When you are pregnant, ideally, you have your provider checking in and helping you through each month of your pregnancy. However, during the fourth trimester, most women are on their own. You may have a checkup or two; otherwise, you are navigating a significant life change left to your own devices. A postpartum doula will help you adapt to life with your newborn for days, weeks, or months—however long you need.

A good doula is like your fairy Godmother sent from the birthing and postpartum heavens. Many people know about birth doulas and how they help decrease long labor, decrease C-section rates, and improve overall experiences for mamas in labor (Bancoff, 2018). They held your hair back as you puked, pushed on your back for hours, and encouraged you when you did not think you could continue. Imagine having someone come to your home and continue that support!

Instead of loading everyone up in the car, time the pumping and nursing, pack the diaper bag—you get the idea. It is a lot! Postpartum doulas are a game-changer!

Doulas understand what new mothers go through as their hormones fluctuate. They can help with practical tasks, too, like meal prep and helping you comfortably breastfeed. They focus on the new mother's physical and mental health while encouraging a strong bond between mother and baby.

While a doula will not replace your provider, they provide support in many ways you will not get from your regular checkups (Schneider, 2022). Admittedly for many people, it can be cost-prohibitive. If you have many supplies you need from a previous child or friends and family, ask for money to pay a doula instead of baby shower gifts. People will love knowing they are helping you get what you need to care for yourself and your newborn baby in the fourth trimester, so it is worth the investment. A good doula is worth their weight in gold! There are also some volunteer doula programs out there, and some states are starting to cover doula services, such as California and patients who have Medi-Cal (California Department of Health Care Services, n.d.). Medical-Flex, or other pretax medical "flexible spending accounts" (FSAs) may also cover doula services. While it might only save some tax dollars, a tiny bit saved here and there to help pay for your doula is worth looking into. **BeHerVillage.com** is a fantastic online community that can help with birth and postpartum support through "shower gifts ." Your newborn will not be upset that you registered for support instead of another pack of onesies.

INTERACTIVE ELEMENT

You have learned a lot about the fourth trimester and the importance of self-care during this period. Now, take some time to reflect on what you expect regarding postpartum self-care and new motherhood. Many women write down extensive birth plans but overlook entirely the fourth trimester.

Start by thinking of three areas where you can be kinder to yourself. You might want to write about how you will give yourself the compassion to rest when necessary or to understand when you have had enough and need to focus on yourself while someone else tends to the baby. You can write about how you will cope when feeling overwhelmed or adapt to the lack of routine a newborn often involves.

If you have trouble thinking of ideas for great compassion, consider using some of these sentence starters to get your imagination rolling.

- Today, I am proud that I...
- My body impresses me because...
- I am grateful for...
- I smiled today because...

- If I could do anything for myself, it would be… (and then do it!)

KEY TAKEAWAYS

The fourth trimester can feel unexpected to many new mothers who thought giving birth would be the last big hurdle in pregnancy. All the focus of our society is centered around the birth. People talk about when will the baby be here, where they are giving birth, do they have a birth plan. And then the baby arrives, everyone sends many congratulatory texts, and all the attention and excitement abruptly halt. And it is at that moment that one of the most challenging chapters of parenting begins. Knowing what to expect postpartum can better prepare you to take care of yourself in the way you deserve.

- Self-care is crucial in this period. You must focus on the basics: rest, nutrition, and support.
- Social support comes in many forms, like your partner taking over newborn care when you need to rest, trusted friends and loved ones helping you and the baby, and interaction with other new moms experiencing something similar.
- There are many myths and misconceptions about pregnancy, childbirth, and the postpartum period. If you are unsure about the validity of a statement or advice, ask your provider, trusted friends, and do

your research to ensure you are getting accurate
information.

- A doula can provide support as you navigate the
  emotional and physical changes of the postpartum
  period. They can also help with your newborn and
  handle tasks around the house to make the transition
  easier.

Taking time to think about the postpartum period and your
expectations for that time can help you be kinder to yourself.
As you will learn in the next chapter, self-compassion is
crucial for your well-being.

2

THE HAPPY MAMA'S PATH TO SELF-COMPASSION AND EMOTIONAL RESILIENCE

You don't have to control your thoughts. You just have to stop letting them control you.

— DAN MILLMAN

One of the easiest ways to practice self-compassion is to understand that your thoughts are just that—thoughts. They are not necessarily your reality. You don't even have to take steps to control them through meditation or positive thinking, though you may find those practices helpful. You just need to ensure you don't give them the power to control you, whether it's how you act, react, or feel mentally and emotionally. Keeping the right perspective in your mindset can help you feel emotionally resilient and compassionate toward yourself.

REFLECTING ON YOUR PREGNANCY AND BIRTH STORY

Before you stride toward self-compassion, take some time to reflect on your pregnancy and birth story. What is the first thing women do when they hear you're pregnant? Immediately talk about their pregnancy and birth! It's almost universal! You will be reflecting on this for your entire life. Looking back at this time can help you assess your situation and understand the root cause of many of your thoughts during the postpartum period. You can mentally reflect or write down your observations in a journal—whatever feels the most natural to you and helps you process these experiences.

First, think about your pregnancy. Did it go as you planned? When you were younger, did you envision pregnancy a certain way? When you found out you were pregnant, did you have any expectations? Did your situation align with those thoughts? Is it a good thing that they did or didn't?

Next, think about your delivery. Did it go the way you planned? Did you have a birth plan, and were you able to follow it? If so, was it what you imagined it would be? If not, how do you feel about the reality of childbirth? Processing your birth is so important. I love to open the chart with my patients and show them the notes in their delivery record. Was it smooth and fast? Were there only three sutures when it seemed like a million? Going over this is very helpful to patients. Perhaps they were so tired that they did not know what was happening around them. Alternatively, something they forgot about may have been the coolest thing ever!

Now, dig a bit deeper into your memories of the delivery. Was the actual birth something you thought about, or did you brush it off and try to forget it after you held your baby? Did something appalling happen that keeps replaying itself in your memory? Birth trauma is real, so addressing it is very important for your mental health.

Take time to think about your birth story, whether you write it out or relive it in your memory. Try to focus on every moment you remember. Put yourself back in that place— how did you feel in each instance? How did you feel before you went into labor? Do you remember the contractions? Do you remember the first time you felt or held your baby? What emotions do you associate with your birth story? Do they align with the emotions you hoped to feel from the experience? What's different between your expectations and reality?

Regardless of the overall emotions associated with your birth story, you need to take time to think about it all.

Childbirth is a major life experience, so you should feel comfortable taking time to process it all. Despite countless women giving birth every day, much less throughout history, it can be one of the most unique experiences in the world. You should not write off your birth story as average, normal, or unimportant if it went according to plan. Similarly, you don't need to dwell on it and catastrophize it if it did not go according to plan. Taking time to sit with it and process it at a reality-based level can greatly help you handle the emotions and move forward with self-compassion.

TWELVE TIPS FOR LOVING YOURSELF AS A NEW MOM

You have been through many changes in the last nine months to a year, so accepting yourself as a new mom can feel daunting. You may feel mentally, emotionally, and physically unlike yourself. Acknowledge that growing a human and keeping them alive is your new superpower! Give yourself credit where credit is due! You did it! You are that powerful! There are not enough awards, trophies, celebrations, plaques, ribbons, and medals in the world to honor what you have accomplished! These tips will help you accept this new version of yourself and love yourself for all you are, celebrating those accomplishments.

- **Try to accept everything.** It can feel insurmountable to function some days, but you should accept the state of things without feeling like you need to change it. If you feel overwhelmed and need to cry, cry. If you're having a good day, enjoy it instead of worrying about what may come tomorrow. It is okay to feel the feels!

- **Make time for yourself.** It's tough to suddenly have a newborn in your care, especially with society making mothers feel like they must give their babies their entire selves. You should not feel guilty about making time for yourself. Whether sipping a cup of tea while it's still hot or soaking in an Epsom salt bath to soothe your body, make time to be alone and enjoy yourself.

- **Breathe fresh air.** You may think you should always stay close to your baby during these first few months, but getting fresh air can make a huge difference in your demeanor and outlook. Leave your baby with your partner or a loved one and take a slow, enjoyable walk around the neighborhood. You can even take a lap around the block or meander through your yard or a nearby park. If you don't have someone to watch your little one, bring them with you so you both benefit from fresh air and some time outside of the house.

- **Cuddle your baby.** Physical connection is a great way to bond with your baby and feel content. You may not want to hold your baby all the time, which can get tiring, but making quality time for cuddles will help you and your baby develop a strong, loving relationship. Acknowledge that you are everything that your baby needs. You are your baby's safe place. You are amazing for that!

- • **Treasure the small moments.** It's easy to feel overwhelmed by the never-ending to-do list of being a parent, so it's crucial to treasure the small moments you might otherwise overlook. Think about yourself and what you like to do with your time, and find small instances throughout the day where you can enjoy those activities. Instead of cleaning the kitchen while the baby naps, kick back on the couch and read a few chapters of the latest page-turner you could not wait to get your hands on. Or simply veg out and let your mind wander without worries.

- **Prioritize nutrition.** This tip may not sound as fun as other self-care options on the list, but it has a lot of power to make you feel great, which is crucial for self-acceptance and compassion. Treating your body right by giving it the nutrition it craves will make it be kinder to you in return, ensuring you have the necessary fuel to care for yourself and your baby in the ways you deserve.

- **Utilize your support network.** Though it can feel intimidating to ask for help, it's better to ask and receive more than you expected than to struggle to make it through the day. You know who you can trust with your postpartum care and your newborn, so reach out to those people when you need a helping hand. You will feel much better about yourself when you don't feel alone, so that self-compassion may come more easily.

- **Socialize.** Reaching out for help is not the only reason to contact your support network. Call or text someone to chat. You'll feel more connected and get back in touch with who you were before giving birth. You can talk about the baby and motherhood, or you can talk about the latest episode of your favorite show—whatever feels right and helps you connect with others.

- **Communicate with your partner.** It's too easy to focus on your baby and let yourself and your partner fall back on your list of priorities. It may feel tough to balance all these relationships during the fourth trimester, but they can make you feel amazing. Communicating with your partner will help you care for yourself because you feel connected and supported. Keeping the lines of communication open can also help you and your partner find your parenting groove.

- **Marvel at your progress.** While new parenthood may feel like a never-ending to-do list, make time to reflect on all you have accomplished. A year ago, you may never have imagined that you would be here, recovering from childbirth and holding your newborn. You are Wonder Woman, and your body and spirit are amazing! After giving birth, you should feel a sense of accomplishment with every bit of progress you make each day. This stage of life can feel daunting, but you should be proud of how you're making it through!

- **Feel gratitude.** Even when you're overwhelmed and feel like the baby won't nap soon enough, give yourself the space to feel gratitude about your life. It doesn't matter if you're crying at the kitchen table—feel grateful for where you are and how you got there. Things will continue to change, so appreciating every moment will bring you a sense of peace, providing a strong foundation for self-compassion.

- **Be patient.** Despite what you see in pop culture or on social media, it is not an instant fix to bounce back to who you were before pregnancy. It can be a long road to recovery, and feeling impatient about where you are compared to where you wish you were will only bring you down. Give yourself the gift of patience to make progress at your pace, however gradual that may be. You have been through something major and should not feel pressure—from yourself or outside sources—to speed up the process or become a certain person by the end of it. Try not to focus on the end result; instead, take time and patience to enjoy the journey.

THE ROLE OF SELF-COMPASSION

Many people think they're good to their friends because they support their social circle, listen to them, help them through the hard times, and celebrate with them during the good times. However, those same people rarely give themselves the same grace. They may be the kindest person in the world… to others! But to themselves, they are much harsher. One of the easiest ways to start practicing self-compassion is to treat yourself like you would treat a friend.

If your friend just had a baby, would you eye her up and down and tell her to get on the treadmill? No way! So, why would you tell yourself to do that? Remember the rotisserie chicken trick? Asking them to leave it at the front door? What if your neighbor friend who just had a baby asked you to grab one while you're at Costco? Most likely, you would!

Many people are their own worst critics. It may be good in certain situations, like pushing yourself to complete a work project or training for a marathon. But you don't want a critic when it comes to postpartum recovery—you *need* a support system. You can support yourself with self-compassion.

Studies show that new mothers who practice self-compassion feel less guilt in terms of taking time for themselves, away from the baby, and motherhood (Bean et al., 2022). Therefore, self-compassion can improve your psychological health. When you feel less guilt for prioritizing self-care, you feel better overall. You may feel happier, healthier, and more energetic. With this refreshed sense of self, new mothers are more likely to increase their physical activity, helping them stay active and healthy while boosting their emotional and mental states.

HOW CAN YOU INCREASE SELF-COMPASSION?

The best way to increase self-compassion is to treat yourself like your best friend. Before you think a mean thought about yourself, stop and imagine saying it to your best friend. If you would never, then stop the thought. If it's not appropriate for a friend, it is not appropriate for you.

Accept yourself where you are without pushing yourself to make progress or change. Be patient and take every day as it comes. In fact, sometimes, taking it "one day at a time" may be too much. Let's just see how the next 15 minutes go. Also, refrain from comparing yourself to other mothers, whether you know them in person or see them online. You can change if you want to, but there's no urgency to do it now while healing and adjusting to parenthood.

Above all, remember that humans are imperfect. What you see on social media is not real. People rarely show the reality of their lives because they want to put their best side forward, which is fine, as long as you realize that and don't compare yourself to an impossible state. Everyone has struggles and difficulties, so don't feel down because you're having a hard time. It's natural and will pass eventually, but giving yourself grace in the meantime can help it feel a little easier to manage.

This may sound silly to some people, but when I'm feeling sad or bad about myself and wish I could look, be, act, or live like some superstar, I try to picture them having diarrhea. Everyone has had diarrhea in their life, and it is certainly not glamorous! It just brings my brain back to the reality that we are all humans.

If you find yourself feeling down, try not to wallow in those feelings. Once you start, it is too easy to feel like you are drowning in that negativity. However, overcompensating with toxic positivity can be just as detrimental. It's best to allow yourself to feel emotions without getting too attached to them. Always envision the big picture without getting overwhelmed by the small moments.

Mindfulness and Relaxation

You can increase self-compassion by practicing mindfulness and making time for relaxation.

Mindfulness is a way to calm yourself and reduce anxiety. You pace yourself by taking time to pay attention to the present without worrying about the future or thinking about the past (Anxiety Canada, n.d.). You allow yourself to experience whatever is currently happening without trying to judge or analyze it—just living in the moment. You take note of everything going on, so you are fully engaged with the experience. For example, if you are in your yard, you are taking deep breaths to appreciate how the fresh air feels in your lungs. You're noticing the colors and scents of the flowers around you. You feel the grass beneath your feet and hear a neighbor mowing the grass a few houses away. You're not thinking that the sound is loud or that it reminds you that you need to cut your lawn—you are only in the moment, accepting everything around you.

Feeling anxious is the opposite of mindfulness. You're worried about what may happen in the future. You are dwelling on something that happened in the past. These thoughts make you anxious even though you cannot do anything about it. All you have is this moment, so appreciating it for what it is helps you stay mindful and connected.

Some anxiety can be a good thing, so don't beat yourself up if you sometimes feel anxious. Anxiety can be a tool to keep us safe, like looking both ways when crossing a street or putting our seatbelts on in the car. It caused some form of anxiety in our lives, and now it has turned into a habit, and most likely, the anxiety of crossing the street or feeling safer when you drive is gone.

Being mindful can help you relax, but there are other techniques to calm down, too. The goal is to refocus attention from something stressful to something calming. You should become more aware of your body to stay positive and help solve problems.

Autogenic relaxation is a way to use visuals and awareness to calm down. Think of an image or phrase that helps you calm down, and repeat it to yourself. As the action helps you relax, take steps to release your muscle tension, regulate your breathing, and feel all sensations in your body.

Progressive muscle relaxation is another way to calm down. You focus on each muscle group in your body, thinking of it, feeling it, and letting it go to release stress. You can start at your toes and work up, or vice versa. Tense the muscles as you think of them, then release them and move on to the next group. Similarly, yoga, tai chi, massage, and deep breathing can help you become more aware of your body and relax (Mayo Clinic, 2017). Some great apps, like Calm, Headspace, and Insight Timer, can help with guided imagery or stories to help calm your body down.

Relaxation takes practice, so give yourself time and patience to explore these methods. Consider adding a few of these one-minute practices from Psych Central (2021) into your day.

- **Sit.** Yes, sit for one minute, with good posture, without being too stiff. Keep your feet flat on the floor and rest your hands on your thighs. Close your eyes and focus on your breath entering and leaving your body. Start with one minute, but continue the practice as long as you can. When you are done, gradually open your eyes, reorient yourself with your surroundings, and return to your day.

- **Walk.** You can walk around the neighborhood, from the porch to your car or even from your bedroom to the kitchen. Pay attention to each step you take. How many steps do you take for each inhale or exhale? Does your breath impact your walking speed? Do not force your breath or your pace; just notice everything. As you walk, you can match your steps to your breath, counting "one, two, three" as you move your body and feel like you're completely in tune with yourself.

- **Box breathing.** You can do this meditation anytime you have a free minute. As you inhale, count to four and visualize the top of a box. Hold your breath as you count to four and picture one side of the box. Exhale while you count to four and visualize the bottom of the box. Hold your breath again, counting to four and visualizing the final side of the box. Do this as many times as you need to feel calm and centered.

- **Free-range meditation.** You can practice this meditation with any daily task. For example, if you're taking a shower, think about each thing as you do it. When you turn on the water, pay attention to the temperature and how it feels on your body and sounds to your ears. Feel each stream from the shower head. Change the temperature and stay present in how it feels. You can even continue feeling the sensations and staying present as you dry off and get dressed, ready to face your day. Try doing this when you eat meals, brush your teeth, or do other daily tasks and see how it roots you and helps you feel connected to your life.

Over time, you will realize how much the benefits of relaxation can impact you. You will be able to slow your heart rate and lower your blood pressure. You can improve digestion and regulate your blood sugar levels. The ability to relax means you're able to reduce stress hormones and decrease muscle tension which can lead to chronic pain. As a result, you'll sleep better, boost your focus, and improve your mood (Mayo Clinic, 2017).

Support Groups

Support groups can help you relax and practice self-compassion because you get together with people in similar situations. Hearing about what other new moms experience helps you realize that your issues are normal, and you should not feel bad about how you make it through the day. Support groups also give you a chance to get advice from people who have been there and done that or are currently going through it too. With this type of communication, you have a great chance of making new friends. Connecting with people in a similar stage of life is a good way to stay more in touch with who you are and whom you can become without feeling the stress of comparing yourself to others. It offers accountability because you can relate to these mothers and talk about how you're feeling and what benchmarks you're reaching.

You can also achieve personal growth through a support group. You have people meeting you where you are and accepting that, so you will also accept yourself while still realizing your full potential. You will feel more secure, which will inspire you to make changes and reach goals on your timeline instead of comparing yourself to unattainable lives you may see on social media.

The term "support groups" may make you think of a new mom group, but that's just one way you can find support. Your partner, parents, siblings, and family can be a support group. Your friends can provide support. Your coworkers can provide support, even when you are on parental leave. New parents and related groups can definitely provide support. However, other communities can, too, like people at the library or regulars you see at your favorite cafe and enjoy small talk with, alleviating some of your stress. There are many types of support, so accepting it where you can find it will greatly benefit your mental and emotional health.

Realistic Expectations

You already know how I feel about society's expectations of new mothers. It's as if you're supposed to be a magical superhero, bouncing back to your original body and energy levels while also caring for a new baby, thinking nothing of all the pain you went through to get here. The lack of postpartum care and adequate parental leave is another story—how can you be the fully invested mother society expects if you have to go right back to work to make ends meet?

However, there is a delicate balance between harsh reality and unrealistic expectations. Thinking you should be a superhero can make you feel depressed and inadequate. But the harsh reality of postpartum care can make you feel depressed and angry. The best solution is to balance your expectations to be what you can realistically handle without concerning yourself with what others may think.

You may hear different, often contradictory things from people when you're pregnant and have a newborn. Someone may say that motherhood comes naturally and babies are delightful, but you feel it's a struggle to adapt to your new role, and your baby is cranky more than they seem happy. Another person may say your life won't change once you have a baby, but you feel overwhelmed with the new sleep schedule and how baby toys took over your living room.

This section could be a list of myths relating to pregnancy and new parenthood. Do not get me started on people who say pregnancy is wonderful and fulfilling, making you glow from the inside out. In reality, women may experience prenatal depression just as they can have postpartum depression. They may feel like a different being took over their body instead of feeling fulfilled. They may be sweating and not glowing; thank you very much!

It's easy to let these sayings get to you, but most people say them with good intentions. It can feel frustrating to smile and nod, but it's best to let these unrealistic expectations roll off your back. Do not let anyone's cliches impact what you are feeling. You should have your own expectations in mind, and you can talk about them with your partner or someone you trust. Be open about your feelings during pregnancy and the fourth trimester. Talk about the kind of parent you want to be and how you want your baby to fit into your lifestyle. And if they keep trying to shove it down your throat, smile at them, showing both rows of teeth, and then tell them you have to excuse yourself to change your Tucks pad out. That typically will stop a conversation!

It's easy to want to be a stay-at-home mom creating the most fun play stations and cutest snacks for her children, but that may not be you. If you love your job, or even if you don't but need to work to make ends meet, you shouldn't also feel like you need to make gourmet lunch boxes for your child to take to daycare. And there is no shame in sending your kid to daycare—you have to be realistic about what you want and need for your life and strive to make those expectations your reality.

I learned that I'm not a good full-time worker with kids, but I also learned that I'm not a good full-time mom and need to have work in my life as well. And I am 100% okay with that! Maybe my confidence in that grew with the birth of each of my children because it did get easier over time with the mental ping-pong game going on in my head.

An additional point that can be very stressful to new moms is how the baby is fed. Our expectations can be very different than our reality. I find that there is so much pressure to breastfeed that we sometimes lose sight of what we are trying to achieve, which is a healthy momma and healthy baby. This section could certainly be a book on its own! Breastfeeding is really hard! Babies may come out with the reflexes to nurse, but it is still a learned activity for both baby and mom. While there are many reasons to breastfeed, there can also be just as many reasons why someone doesn't. And this is okay! I know countless stories of moms who worked and worked at nursing, tried all that they could, spent countless hours with lactation specialists, spent hundreds of dollars on equipment and supplements and it still did not work for them. I want to hug all those parents and tell them that it is just fine if they want to stop. Chest, breast, pumping, bottle, formula; Fed is best. This should not be a reflection of our self-worth but rather a choice, that is sometimes made for us, and to be ok with this decision. And while it may work fine for many, the expectation that all babies can be perfectly chest/breastfed is not fair and unrealistic.

How to Add Self-Care To Your Routine

It might seem like you already have so much on your plate that adding self-care is a step too far. In that case, you should know that doing less is okay. Don't push yourself to make every day the best day—sometimes, making it through only crying five times is a victory! You should trust yourself instead of doubting every action and feeling like you need verification from another person or the internet. Care for yourself by doing what you need to get by without trying to be perfect. Oh, and take tons of pictures because this time flies, and you may have trouble remembering it since you're so consumed in the moment. You can never have too many pictures of your little one. During this time, you will be creating a strong bond with your child, and that should be more important than keeping the house clean or scrolling unattainably cute photos on social media.

You can add self-care into your routine without feeling like you're taking on more work. Simple steps count as self-care and can make you feel better than you expect. For example, drinking plenty of water and eating when you're hungry will help you feel satisfied and healthy, boosting your energy levels and improving your sleep patterns. You can get even more rest by napping when your baby does, which is absolutely a form of self-care! You don't have to insert new things into your schedule to add self-care. Just see what you can fit into your existing moments to carve out time for yourself.

Make time to be alone throughout the day. Even taking an extra five minutes to close yourself in the bathroom, even if you're not soaking in the tub, can help you clear your mind and reduce some of your stress. You can also socialize, sharing your thoughts and feelings with your partner, friends, family, or support group. Asking these people for help can also free up some time for self-care.

Remember that self-care does not have to mean you say yes to something, like going on a walk or meeting a friend for coffee. Self-care can mean saying no. If someone wants to visit, but you don't have the capacity for guests, say no. That is self-care because you are listening to yourself and what you want. Saying no to housework can also be a way to take care of yourself, protecting your time and energy.

INTERACTIVE ELEMENT

Thinking about what can help you cope with the hard times will ensure you navigate those situations without letting stress and anxiety take over. Fill out this worksheet, really thinking about what will make you feel better when you're depressed, stressed, or anxious. Keep it handy so you can read it when you're overwhelmed and better handle the hard moments of the day.

The left column of this worksheet explains the six coping skills. Read about each one and, in the right column, write examples of ways you can use this skill to alleviate your anxiety (Ackerman, 2017).

Coping skill	My strategy
Thought challenging: Acknowledge, confront, and dispute thoughts that make you feel uncertain or depressed.	
Releasing emotions: What activity can give you an outlet for your emotions?	
Practicing self-care: What are some ways you can practice self-care and show yourself love or take time to relax? What activities will energize you when you need it? What will calm you down when you're anxious?	
Distracting: Sometimes, you can't face your negative thoughts or difficult experiences, so it's best to distract yourself before they make you spiral. How can you distract yourself to prevent depression?	
Finding your best self: What core beliefs do you have that you don't think you're expressing at the moment? How can you get in touch with your truest self and let that goodness shine through?	
Grounding: How can you center yourself in the current moment, letting go of any worries about the past or future? What thoughts will help you feel connected to the present?	

KEY TAKEAWAYS

Knowing that postpartum parents need self-care and understanding what steps to take to reach that situation are two drastically different ideas. This chapter helped you understand what you can do to take care of yourself as you heal from childbirth.

- Reflect on your pregnancy and childbirth experience. So many mothers feel the need to move on to keep their heads above water, but making time to think about what you went through can help you neutralize the past and empower you to move forward.
- You have undergone so many changes throughout pregnancy, childbirth, and now in postpartum. It's too easy to wish you looked a different way or felt like someone else, but the tips for self-love in this chapter can help you appreciate who you are right now.
- Self-compassion means you are kind to yourself, just as you would treat a friend. Changing your approach may take some trial and error, but the results are major benefits that help you feel mentally and emotionally at the top of your game.
- There are many ways to integrate self-compassion into your life, like practicing mindfulness, making time to relax, relying on support groups, and having realistic expectations for yourself and parenthood.
- Choosing how you feed your baby is not a reflection of your self-worth.
- Adding self-care to your routine does not require a scheduling overhaul—find moments for yourself and

allow yourself to take time to relax and stay calm without the mom guilt.

- Remember that this newborn time is just a phase—your life will keep changing, and your baby will grow. There is much to look forward to, so don't feel overwhelmed. As you will see in the next chapter, understanding perinatal mood and anxiety disorders can empower you to handle them without feeling like you have lost yourself.

BEYOND THE BABY BLUES— PERINATAL MOOD AND ANXIETY DISORDERS

One in five women experiences a perinatal mood and anxiety disorder (PMAD) after childbirth (The Motherhood Center of New York, 2022). Since the pandemic, those numbers have been on the rise, but almost 80% of the cases are undiagnosed. Sometimes it's because of the stigma associated with PMAD, lack of awareness, or the inability to find treatment options.

This chapter could be a 1,000-page novel in itself! There is so much to say in this day and age regarding mental health, specifically mental health regarding pregnancy and postpartum. We will have more accurate statistics in years to come, but I have seen a significant increase in this subject. More so coming out of a pandemic. It has become progressively more and more common. Understanding the symptoms can empower you to take control of your overall well-being during the fourth trimester.

DISTINGUISHING TYPICAL POSTPARTUM CHANGES FROM CONCERNING SYMPTOMS

Most moms experience some sort of change after childbirth, whether it's the relatively tolerable baby blues, involving mood swings and crying spells, or something more debilitating, like postpartum depression. Understanding the differences between these two situations can help you stay aware of what you are going through. Knowing what you feel and how to handle it can make a major difference in your healing process, your self-care, and how you parent your newborn.

Regardless of what you are going through, there is no shame in baby blues or postpartum mood disorders. It is something natural that can happen after you give birth. It is not a character flaw or a sign that you are not fit to be a parent—it's simply a complication you may face after giving birth. You can seek help in these situations to ensure you have support and get treatment that helps you feel like yourself again, freeing you up to bond with your baby.

Baby Blues

Society makes it seem like new parents are absolutely elated at the birth of their baby. However, going through childbirth is a hefty feat for both mother and baby, even if you were able to follow your dream birth plan. It can be easy for some and debilitating for others. Both bodies underwent a major change, and it's a shock to the system, so you shouldn't feel like you need to bounce right back, physically or mentally (Mayo Clinic, 2018b).

Some common symptoms of baby blues include

- worries or anxiety
- appetite problems
- crying spells
- feeling overwhelmed
- focusing issues
- irritability
- mood swings
- sleep problems

You may experience mild symptoms of baby blues, which many new mothers expect, and an average of 75% experience (Cleveland Clinic, 2022a). After all, your body just went through something incredible and amazing, yet painful. You are trying to physically heal from that while also adapting to caring for a newborn. It's not surprising that you'll be unable to get much sleep. And with your hormones all over the place, of course, you will have mood swings! Sometimes it just feels like too much, which leads to crying spells. You might have severe symptoms, meaning you spend most of your time fluctuating between the signs above while doing what is necessary to care for your newborn, but otherwise, you are not living life to its fullest.

I like to tell people that all bets are off for the first two weeks. You may not know what day it is; peek out the window to see if the sun is up or down. You gauge time by when the baby last ate. But after that, the clouds should start to part. You may even put a shirt on that's not inside out!

The good thing to note is that this feeling is temporary. Baby blues are feelings mothers most commonly feel two or three days after giving birth, once the euphoria of being Wonder Woman wears off. You can feel these symptoms for up to two weeks, but you adapt to your new situation at that point, and the baby blues go away. If they don't go away, you may be dealing with something more severe.

Postpartum Depression and Anxiety

About 15% of women experience postpartum depression after giving birth (Cleveland Clinic, 2022a). It might feel like the baby blues, but it is more severe and does not go away after a few weeks. It can happen anytime in the first year— not necessarily after the immediate postpartum period. At that point, you should seek treatment through counseling, medication, or both to help overcome this obstacle. The earlier the interventions the better.

Many new parents struggle to identify what they're feeling. After all, your life just changed drastically. Sure, pregnancy may give you some time to prepare, but whatever you were expecting, the reality is most likely going to be different. Even after carrying a baby for nine, ten, or more months, holding the little human in your arms gives you an entirely different feeling. Most mothers dream of giving birth, feeling their new baby in their arms, and immediately falling in love. Sometimes that can happen. Sometimes mothers don't feel that connection, either because they're still trying to process the birth or, you know, they don't fall in love with someone they met two minutes ago!

Okay, I am joking about making light of the situation, but seriously, there is no shame in not falling head over heels for your tiny, wrinkly brand-new baby instantly. Think of how society reacts to new fathers—they're rarely expected to feel love for their newborn immediately. They are given time to process the change and get to know this new person before they fall in love (Vinopal, 2022). Many people argue that mothers have the months of pregnancy to bond with their baby, but again, this isn't always the case. You are so busy keeping this human alive inside your body, getting the necessary supplies, and nesting that you might not have had the time to feel connected in utero. Even if you did, meeting the baby outside of the womb, when they're likely crying and screaming and immediately thrust into your arms, isn't exactly the sweet "running across a field in slow motion to meet in a loving embrace" first meeting you dream of.

My point is that it can be normal not immediately to feel connected to your baby. You might not feel comfortable holding them. You might have issues breastfeeding. You might just wish they'd close their mouth for one second so you can get some sleep after being in labor for 24 hours! It's normal, seriously. You might feel this irritability for a day. You might feel baby blues for a couple of weeks. But if the feeling persists, it is could be postpartum depression. Do not feel ashamed—just get help immediately. If you are unable to care for yourself, you cannot care for your baby as well, so this is not something you should put off.

There are multiple risk factors for postpartum depression that you may feel during pregnancy or after childbirth (MGH Center for Women's Mental Health, 2015). They can include

1. Prenatal depression
2. Prenatal anxiety
3. Previous depressive episodes
4. Maternity blues
5. Stressful life events
6. Inadequate social support
7. Poor marital relationship
8. Low self-esteem
9. Stress regarding childcare
10. Difficult temperament in your infant
11. Doing it on your own/single
12. Unplanned or unwanted pregnancy
13. Low socioeconomic status
14. Pregnancy complications
15. Mothers whose infants are in the NICU
16. Mothers of multiples

17. Mothers who have gone through infertility treatments
18. Women with any form of diabetes

In many cases, your provider may note that you meet some of these variables during your pregnancy, and they will prepare you for what may come after giving birth. They can monitor you closely to ensure you feel empowered and supported along the way. Early intervention can prepare you for what may come, so you get help before it reaches a point where you can hardly bear it (MGH Center for Women's Mental Health, 2015).

Symptoms of postpartum depression can resemble baby blues initially. You'll cry. You'll go through mood swings. You'll feel irritable. Nevertheless, that is where the similarities end (Fulghum Bruce, 2003).

If you have experienced depression before, you may recognize the signs. You may feel helpless and hopeless. You may struggle to bond with your baby and start to distance yourself from family and friends. You may lose sleep and go through appetite changes, eating too much or not enough. These factors all impact your energy, so you'll feel overwhelmingly fatigued. This can pile on and possibly make you feel like you're a terrible mother. Since you cannot think straight due to lack of sleep and food and this new being in your midst, you may feel frustrated that you cannot seem to make decisions. These symptoms might lead to panic attacks. It can even progress to the point where you think about harming yourself or your newborn (Mayo Clinic, 2018b).

Placental corticotropin-releasing hormone (pCRH) levels increase during the third trimester of pregnancy. A major increase in pCRH can predict the likelihood and severity of postpartum depression (Mikulak & Wolpert, 2013). Despite the prevalence of hormones in this research, the study also found that social and emotional support improved the mother's overall well-being. They felt secure and understood instead of anxious and struggling, which eased the transition into motherhood (Negron et al., 2013). Sadly, there is no magic blood draw to predict how each individual will react or feel. Or a formula to see how your experience will be. But this does show that social and emotional support was a game changer.

This paragraph hints at what you may feel—it's not the definitive set of experiences you will face as a new parent. Most mothers can't pinpoint the exact thing that feels off. They will tell me, "I just don't feel like myself." Or "I don't know who I am." They may not be able to identify any of the symptoms in the previous paragraph, even if it's what they're going through. They feel...different. They think it is their new identity, whom they are meant to be as a mother, so they may not notice how down they feel and how they're meeting many symptoms of postpartum depression.

Postpartum depression can last for several months or even longer, so it is crucial that you get treatment as soon as you recognize the symptoms. If you do not recognize it yourself, listen to your loved ones. Your partner, friends, or parents may notice that you seem different after giving birth. It can be difficult to listen to them talk about your state of being, but you should trust them if you don't see it in yourself. They are your support system and want what's best for you.

That said, sometimes situations do not resolve themselves neatly. For example, I was not diagnosed with postpartum depression until five or six months after giving birth. I thought what I was going through was normal—I had a newborn, wasn't I supposed to cry every day? But it was more than that. I felt like I couldn't do anything right, that maybe I wasn't cut out for motherhood. What was this happiness of motherhood people spoke of? Somedays, it seemed like it would be easier to let myself sink beneath the water in the bathtub and just never come up for air, especially since I felt like I was suffocating in real life, too. Thankfully, I was still in touch with my midwife and told her how I felt. She recognized the signs and helped me get the support I needed to come up for air and get past it. So, you may not know about your postpartum depression as quickly as you would expect, which is just one reason why a support system is so crucial.

Postpartum Psychosis

In rare instances, typically in one out of every thousand births, postpartum depression can escalate into postpartum psychosis. You may notice symptoms as early as a week after giving birth, and they can come on strong. You may feel confused or lost in life, possibly even hallucinating and having delusions. You may struggle to sleep and often feel paranoid or obsessive about your baby. You may attempt to hurt yourself or the baby. This condition is incredibly serious, and you should not waste any time getting treatment for the well-being of yourself and your newborn.

These are the horror stories that we see in the media that make us all catch our breath. Seeing these stories can be triggering and cause many emotions in and of themselves. My heart is absolutely crushed when I hear about these. And I also get so mad and angry because I know that in the right circumstances, these cases can be stopped and helped for all involved.

Postpartum psychosis is a medical emergency, with hallucinations and delusions as the most common symptoms. There are also different types of symptoms, such as depressive, manic, and atypical or mixed (Cleveland Clinic, 2022b).

Depressive symptoms make up the most common subgroup of postpartum psychosis, with about 41% of cases displaying this type of symptom (Cleveland Clinic, 2022b). You may feel anxious or panicked along with depression. You may feel guilty and unable to enjoy things you used to love. You may experience delusions, hallucinations, and thoughts of harming yourself or your child, possibly linked with the hallucinations in that you feel commanded to hurt your child or yourself.

Manic symptoms are the second most common, as seen in about 34% of postpartum psychosis cases (Cleveland Clinic, 2022b). The risk of physical harm to your or your child is lower, but you may still experience symptoms like irritability, agitation, aggression, and functioning on less sleep.

Atypical symptoms are about 25% of cases that mix some of the things you may see in depressive and manic situations (Cleveland Clinic, 2022b). You may also feel confused, disoriented, or appear like you are not awake and be unaware of what is going on around you. You may speak strangely and make inappropriate comments or be completely mute.

Postpartum psychosis is more common in people with a history of mental health conditions in themselves or their family background. First-time parents are more likely to experience these symptoms, but it can still happen after subsequent pregnancies. However, other things completely unrelated to your biology can cause postpartum psychosis, such as sleep deprivation and hormone changes (Cleveland Clinic, 2022b).

Anyone feeling this way has a high risk of harming themselves or their children. If you think you have postpartum psychosis, call 911 immediately (Cleveland Clinic, 2022b). The safety of you and your loved ones is most important at this time, but once you are safe, you can get a diagnosis from your provider.

THE IMPORTANCE OF SEEKING PROFESSIONAL HELP FOR POSTPARTUM ISSUES

Treatment can help you manage PMAD symptoms and improve your well-being. When the symptoms become long-term, it progresses into chronic depression. While treatment may make you feel better, you want to continue with help and support, since stopping too early can cause you to relapse.

One method of PMAD treatment is psychotherapy (Mayo Clinic, 2018a). You'll meet with a mental health professional, like a psychologist or licensed clinical social worker, and discuss your feelings and problems. The professional will help you set realistic goals and respond to life situations in a positive way. They can help you build your tool basket of what you can use to get through this. And while mental health care in the U.S. has struggled with access for everyone, many practices are making it a bit easier. There are Zoom meetings, phone call appointments, and apps that can help you check in.

Another treatment option is to take medication. Tell your provider if you are breastfeeding, as the medication can enter your breast milk. However, there are medications you can take that won't cause negative side effects for your baby, so it's worth trying this option to ensure you feel more positive. Your provider may also prescribe anti-anxiety medications or sleeping pills to help you stay calm or get enough rest. They will explain the risks and benefits to you so you can make an informed decision and prioritize your well-being. There is still a stigma in the U.S. for taking medication for mood disorders. And to that, I say shove it! You would never ask a person with diabetes if they could just try a little harder to make insulin. Or have they ever thought about belly breathing through a diabetic crisis? Of course not! And sometimes brain chemicals need some help as well.

If you have an engaged support system, they can also help alleviate issues related to postpartum depression. For example, they can talk to you about your problems and celebrate every win, no matter how small, instead of focusing completely on the baby. Being proactive and helping out instead of asking the mother what she needs is also a powerful way to support people with postpartum depression.

INTERACTIVE ELEMENT

With all the focus on support systems and seeking help, at this stage, you should compile a list of people who can help you. Whom can you call when you are stressed? What is the number for your local crisis center? What are three things you can do when you feel worries mounting and a crisis looming? Think of the meditation and relaxation technique from Chapter 2, plus other methods you have found to calm yourself down.

Making a list helps you feel empowered when these experiences happen. Any time you feel overwhelmed, consult the list and take action.

Friends to call:

Medical/Mental Health Provider:

Urgent help and support:

- National Maternal Mental Health Hotline: Call or text: 1-833-852-6262
- Postpartum Support International Help Line: Call or test: 800-944-4773

Crisis center:

- National Suicide & Crisis Lifeline: Call or text: 988

Ways to alleviate worries:

1.

2.

3.

KEY TAKEAWAYS

Many women experience PMAD but do not get diagnosed or have access to treatment. Some mothers don't even realize what they are going through—they only recognize that they do not feel like themselves. Knowing the symptoms of PMAD can help you advocate for support and treatment.

- Baby blues start a few days after childbirth and can last a few weeks. About 75% of new parents experience this mood disorder, which includes anxiety, crying spells, irritability, mood swings, and sleep issues.
- About 15% of new moms experience postpartum depression and anxiety. It may feel like baby blues but lasts longer and can be more severe. Treatment from a medical professional can help you manage the symptoms with therapy or antidepressants.
- Postpartum psychosis is rare, happening in one of every 1,000 births. It includes hallucinations, delusions, and an increased risk of you hurting yourself or your baby. Those symptoms make this a

medical emergency, so you should seek immediate help.

- Hormone levels can impact your likelihood of experiencing PMAD. However, a solid support system can empower you and help you feel like you can manage the early stages of new parenthood.
- Mental and emotional changes are not all you will navigate in the fourth trimester—you will also notice physical changes. Embracing your new body can greatly help you feel more positive about yourself during this time.

4

THE NEW YOU—PHYSICAL CHANGES AND EMBRACING YOUR NEW MAMA BOD

Postpartum is a quest back to yourself, alone in your body again. You will never be the same; you are stronger than you were.

— AMETHYST JOY

P hysical changes can make it feel like you are not yourself anymore. This feeling makes some new mothers unsettled and uncomfortable with themselves, which may also negatively impact their mental and emotional states. Keeping everything on track in your fourth trimester is a delicate balance, so embracing your new mama bod can significantly impact your overall well-being. So, when you go to wipe for the first time after birth and your perineum is now four inches lower than anticipated, or you have a hemorrhoid that feels like a tree coming out of your bum, or your boobs look like a sack of marbles when your milk comes in—do not panic! This is all temporary, and we can help!

BODY CHANGES AFTER CHILDBIRTH

Your body changes a lot during pregnancy to accommodate your growing baby, so, understandably, it will change even more after giving birth. You may experience discomfort in the perineal area, hemorrhoids, lochia, constipation, pain around your C-section incision, and breast engorgement (Cleveland Clinic, 2018). You can also have vaginal tears from giving birth.

You may feel discomfort in the perineal area, especially if you had an episiotomy. You can sit in a warm sitz bath to alleviate the pain. Clean your perineum whenever you use the bathroom or change your pads using the peri bottle. Squirt the area with warm water and gently pat it dry. You can also soak a pad with witch hazel and pop it in the freezer. Witch hazel is a natural anti-inflammatory, and the frozen aspect will cool your perineum (Motroni, 2023).

Vaginal bleeding after a human comes out of you is expected regardless of whether you had a vaginal delivery or cesarean section. *Lochia* is a discharge that resembles menstrual discharge, appearing dark red for the first few days and possibly including small blood clots. The color looks watered down by the fourth day and may turn brown. By the tenth day, it will turn yellow or cream-colored (Cleveland Clinic, 2018). Wear pads to protect your clothing for four to six weeks after childbirth, when the lochia should end. The more active you are in early postpartum, the longer your bleeding may last.

Many women are very nervous about their tears or lacerations. Remember that this is some of the fastest healing tissue in our body! There is a reason a baby comes out of your vagina and not your belly button! Most people will have more discomfort from a hemorrhoid than a laceration, but everyone is different. Vaginal tears can happen when your tissue cannot accommodate the size or position of the baby exiting your body. Most heal on their own in a few weeks. If the tear needs repairs, you will get stitches, and the sutures will dissolve as the area heals. Second-degree vaginal tears also tear your perineal muscle and will heal with stitches within three or four weeks. Third-degree tears go to the outer capsule of your anal sphincter. You will have to get stitches, and it takes up to six weeks to allow them to heal. Fourth-degree tears are even more severe, going through your sphincter. While not always, you may need to go to the operating room for third- and fourth-degree tears. These can take longer to repair and may need additional equipment to visualize the areas well (Mayo Clinic, n.d.-b). Know that third- and fourth-degree lacerations are not very common.

Take your time in the bathroom! Have a station all set up with your peri bottle, pads, witch hazel, hemorrhoid cream, and clean underwear. You can rinse those mesh panties and use them again while you are in the big mama pads. Save your underwear for later!

You can also relax in a sitz bath at least three days after giving birth. Use warm water and fill the tub two to three inches high to cover your vaginal area. You can use plain water or dissolve Epsom salts in the tub.

This type of bath can also help with hemorrhoid relief. You can have hemorrhoids before childbirth, but many mothers experience them after giving birth. When there is pressure on the veins in your rectum or anus, they weaken and allow blood to pool, causing the area to swell (Johnson, 2023). Hemorrhoids can be one of the most uncomfortable aspects of postpartum. It can feel like a Christmas tree is coming out of your bum, and come to find out; it's only a half-centimeter tissue blob! They can hurt. Most of the time, they will go away on their own, but we do have other things to offer if they do not. You can also eat fiber-rich foods and drink plenty of water to soften your stool and facilitate healthy digestion and bowel movements. Try to walk around or lie down more than you sit to alleviate the pressure on the veins.

You may not have a bowel movement until three or four days after childbirth, and even then, the idea of applying pressure may scare you a bit. Your provider can recommend a stool softener to make the situation more comfortable. You can also eat more fruits and vegetables while drinking at least ten glasses of water to promote a safe, natural bowel movement.

When I do postpartum rounds in the hospital, this is one of the top worries of new mamas! They are very nervous about the first poop! It can be scary, but you will be able to poop! Take your time and go slow. Your body knows to slow peristalsis, or digestion, down in labor, and it will start back up again after the baby is out. This means things will start moving again. Drink, drink, and drink more water! Lots of fiber can help as well. Some medications, especially narcotics, can constipate you, so talk with your provider about this. You can also have urinary incontinence when you leak urine after laughing, sneezing, coughing, jumping, or exercising. You can strengthen your pelvic floor muscles with Kegel exercises to combat this issue. A consult with a pelvic floor physical therapist can be helpful if you continue to have problems with either leaking urine or having a hard time pooping.

- Pooping after birth 101: For vaginal deliveries, you can take a witch hazel pad or tissue, and with that and your hand, gently support your perineum (the area between your vagina and rectum) while having a bowel movement. If you had a C-section, you can take a towel roll or a smaller pillow and support your incision. Having your feet up on a step or Squatty

Potty and gently blowing out your air instead of bearing down hard may be helpful.

Mothers who had a C-section may notice drainage from the incision. You should wash it with soap and water, but if the drainage continues or is not a watery pink, contact your provider for a checkup.

Breast engorgement and discharge are uncomfortable body changes many mothers experience. You can experience engorgement whether you are breastfeeding or bottle-feeding. Your breasts may feel heavy, warm, or hard. Breastfeeding mothers may also feel this symptom if they miss a feeding, so pumping or feeding the baby can alleviate the discomfort. When your breasts are overly full, they will feel swollen, tender, or painful, like they are about to burst. You may even experience a low fever. Prolonged engorgement, or even clogged milk ducts, can lead to a breast infection called Mastitis. This may need to be treated with antibiotics. Contact your provider or a Lactation Consultant if you need help. Sometimes your milk will come in over a day or two, while other times, it may come in like a heavy cement truck ready to dump! I remember my milk coming in and feeling like I had giant golf ball lumps jammed into water balloons that were now attached to my body.

You can take pain medication or apply ice packs to stay comfortable, especially if you are not breastfeeding. You can massage your breasts while feeding your baby or pumping milk. To alleviate the pressure, you can also express a small amount of milk between feedings. It is hard for babies to latch on engorged breasts, so you can take a warm shower to soften your breasts and nipples before feeding. The warm water can alleviate your discomfort, too. Mothers with engorged breasts may notice leakage, so using breast pads will protect your clothing. Breast engorgement is temporary but can continue when you produce milk.

Make sure you have a nursing bra so big you think there is no way you will ever fit in it—because you just might! Trying to squish the girls into a bra that is too small can be uncomfortable and cause medical problems like engorgement or clogged ducts.

CONSEQUENCES OF SLEEP DEPRIVATION POST-PREGNANCY

Sleep deprivation can impact your ability to take care of your newborn. You are not getting enough rest to promote your physical, mental, and emotional health, making everyday tasks much more challenging than they should be. Sleep deprivation can also lead to depression and anxiety. Studies show that new mothers get two hours less sleep than they need, but since they are not getting continuous sleep, that lack is just a small portion of the problem (Hatfield, 2016). A newborn needs about 16 hours of sleep a day but usually only sleeps in bursts of 3 to 4 hours at a time. Since a new mother is often the main source of nutrition for the newborn, they must follow the same schedule. It can be challenging to reach REM sleep in such a short time span, so the mother is not getting quality deep sleep to keep functioning properly.

A lack of sleep can cause decreased energy and exhausting fatigue, which impact your mood and mental well-being (Pacheco & Vyas, 2020). It can seem challenging to distinguish between sleep deprivation and postpartum depression since there is so much overlap in symptoms. Sleep deprivation can exacerbate factors of postpartum depression, so it is tough to pinpoint the cause and effect. With the sudden drop in estrogen, progesterone, and thyroid hormones, your sleep cycle will be interrupted based on those physical changes alone. Add in a newborn sleeping for only three or four hours at a time, and it is hard to get enough rest to remain functional day in and day out.

In addition to the likelihood of depression due to sleep deprivation, the lack of sleep many new mothers experience can also impact their breast milk supply. When you do not get enough sleep, your body produces higher levels of cortisol, which can reduce your milk supply (Hill et al., 2005).

If you need more rest and take on the bulk of care for your newborn, you are putting extra demands on your body. Even though you may feel exhausted, it can feel nearly impossible to quiet your brain enough to get sleep. And then it will feel like you wake up right after you close your eyes without getting the sleep quality necessary for your health. That is where some sleep strategies can come into play to help you make the most of every moment.

Postpartum Sleep Strategies

Living without adequate sleep can feel intolerable, so knowing postpartum sleep strategies can help you get the rest you need. Having a sleep protection plan for the birthing parent is so important! If possible, ask for support from your partner or a postpartum doula. Take shifts so one person can rest while the other handles the baby's needs. If you are breastfeeding, pump and store milk in bottles so someone else can do feedings without needing to wake you up. Ask friends and family to come and be with the baby during the day so you can nap (Johnston, 2021).

Getting sunlight early in the day can help maintain your circadian rhythm, improving your sleep hygiene (Pacheco & Vyas, 2020). Eating a healthy diet and getting appropriate exercise can also help you feel energized while improving your ability to sleep when you have a chance.

The right position can also help you get the best sleep. While we encourage side sleeping during pregnancy, sleeping on your back postpartum can help you get better quality sleep (Olson, 2020). If you have lower back pain while sleeping, put pillows underneath your thighs and lower legs to alleviate the pressure. Your daily habits can also impact your sleep, such as drinking enough fluids and keeping your sodium intake low to reduce swelling so you stay more comfortable when you rest. Keeping your feet elevated when you sit or lie down can also alleviate swelling.

Good sleep hygiene can promote deeper sleep at any time in your life, so it can be especially nice to have a self-care routine to promote sleep during your fourth trimester. Keep your bedroom as dark as possible and make it cool. The darkness and temperature will inspire you to cuddle up and get sleep while remaining comfortable.

Stop using electronics about an hour before you want to go to sleep. Your brain will wind down, and you will not feel kept awake by the light of the screens. You can read a book or magazine but hold a physical copy in your hands instead of reading online. You can also listen to soothing music or meditate. Basic nighttime hygiene routines will also help you mentally and physically prepare for sleep. Take a bath or shower, brush your teeth, wash your face, apply your favorite lotion, and know that these tasks prepare you for restful sleep.

If you are napping throughout the day, setting up this type of routine may be more challenging. After all, it is hard to avoid screens for an hour before sleep if you nap when your baby does! In that case, keeping your bedroom dark and cool can significantly help you fall asleep. You can also avoid caffeine and foods that cause heartburn to ensure you can fall asleep whenever you have a chance.

If you are in bed for over 30 minutes and do not feel yourself falling asleep, you likely will not get any rest at that point (Olson, 2020). Instead of continuing to stay in bed and feel frustrated that you cannot sleep, get up and go into another room. Do not turn on all the lights or brew a pot of coffee—your aim is to still try and get some sleep! Nevertheless, you are just getting a change of scenery, so you do not get more agitated and awake when you are in bed. However, if you feel wide awake, do not force yourself to rest until you feel sleepy again.

Whenever possible, let your partner take nighttime shifts so you can get uninterrupted sleep. Some couples will take a "two and two" schedule, where the mother may wake up and breastfeed the baby as needed for two nights, then the partner wakes up and bottle feeds the baby for the next two nights. Knowing you will get two relatively uninterrupted nights of sleep in a row can make this whole new-parent thing seem much more manageable.

There are other ways to promote "shift work," too. You could do the feedings from 6 p.m. to midnight, and your partner could take midnight to 6 a.m. You can alternate these shifts as necessary, but they will still allow each person to get a fair amount of sleep.

There is no perfect solution for everyone, so try these options in two-week periods. That length of time gives you a chance to see what works for your family and your schedule. You can always try one approach for a month, then move on to something else as the baby starts to sleep more, you get the hang of new parenthood, or you change your schedule in some ways. Trying a sleep strategy does not restrict you to that only, so it is worth attempting many to see what works for you.

How to Treat Postpartum Insomnia

The tips from Chapter 3 about getting rest can help you treat insomnia. Having support and people to ask for help can also give you more time to sleep. Napping when the baby sleeps is another way to know you will get a certain amount of rest per day without worrying about someone watching the baby while you close your eyes. You will hear them when they wake up, so you can rest and feel better for the next period of the day.

Postpartum insomnia can happen due to your hormones or lifestyle changes. With your hormones dropping, your body's circadian rhythm changes and disrupts your natural sleep and wake cycles. You may feel sleepy during the day and awake at night. Of course, your baby being up at random times does not help you stay on a strict schedule. You also have to juggle the stress of being a new parent.

Trying to keep a schedule can significantly help your sleep patterns. Even if your baby wakes up every three hours, you can have a meal schedule that helps your body sense when it is time to wind down for a lengthier sleep in the evening. You will have external cues, like putting away the dinner dishes, to help you understand that it is nighttime on some level. Having support from your partner will help even more, especially if you sleep in shifts and know your sleep period is approaching (Phillips, 2022).

If you continue to have sleep issues for the first few months postpartum, you should talk to your medical provider. Some symptoms can be a normal sign of sleep deprivation related to adjusting to new parenthood and your newborn's schedule. However, it can also be a sign of postpartum depression, so getting help from a professional can make a big difference in your overall well-being (Pacheco & Vyas, 2020).

In most cases, postpartum insomnia improves as your baby starts sleeping for more extended periods through the night. If your baby is sleeping, but you still are not, you may have chronic insomnia instead of postpartum insomnia. You can get help from your provider to ensure you are able to rest, as insomnia can put you at risk when you are driving or caring for your baby. It can also lead to other health problems, like diabetes, hypertension, and obesity (Phillips, 2022). Your provider can help you find a solution that prevents your health from deteriorating due to lack of sleep.

HORMONAL CHANGES AFTER CHILDBIRTH

You can find plenty of books about how your body changes during pregnancy. You can download an app that gives you a week-by-week overview of how your baby grows inside you and your body changes to accommodate that growth. But do you know much about how your body changes after childbirth? Like most aspects of postpartum care, many people overlook this period because the baby is out, and you need to focus on their care—does it matter what your body is going through? Yes! Your body just gave birth to an actual human after growing this baby for nine or ten months! It will not bounce back to what it was a year ago because there is a lot to adjust to and heal from.

Your hormones change during pregnancy and continue to fluctuate for about two months after childbirth (Davis, 2023). An influx of estrogen and progesterone prepares your body for pregnancy, including maintaining the uterine lining and preventing the uterus from delivering your baby too early. Your body also releases oxytocin to produce contractions during labor and prolactin to aid milk production. Once you give birth, you get a rush of oxytocin that promotes bonding with your new baby and makes you feel like Wonder Woman. It is the love hormone! This is that yummy feeling when that baby is tucked in under your chin or when you breathe in how they smell. However, oxytocin can also make you feel anxious because you are worried about your baby's safety. Progesterone naturally balances anxiety, but your body makes less after giving birth. It is frustrating because you are not getting a normal balance of hormones to provide for your overall well-being.

One major hormone shift comes when you deliver the placenta because the estrogen and progesterone it contains leave your body. At the same time, your body produces more oxytocin and prolactin to boost your milk supply. You are also adjusting to relaxin levels, which makes your joints looser during pregnancy to accommodate the baby's growth and the act of childbirth but can continue for several months after delivery to make your body feel unlike yourself. These changes in hormone levels can lead to baby blues and postpartum depression.

Postpartum hair loss is another common issue many women experience. Thankfully, the American Academy of Dermatology Association specifies that this is not true hair loss—it is excessive shedding due to your dropping estrogen levels. It is a temporary problem, and your hair will most likely return to its pre-pregnancy state by your baby's first birthday. But if you want to lessen the impact of your hair loss, you can use a volumizing shampoo and conditioner to make your hair look fuller. Avoid "conditioning shampoos" or anything not labeled for fine hair, as these products will coat your strands and make them look limp. You can apply conditioner to only the ends of your hair to prevent it from weighing down the hair on your scalp. You may even want to try a new hairstyle, trusting the stylist to help your hair look full and fresh.

The Hormonal Component of "Baby Blues" and Postpartum Depression

It can feel daunting to understand the hormonal aspect of baby blues and postpartum depression because many people think it is a natural occurrence due to giving birth and adjusting to a drastically different lifestyle and schedule as a new parent. However, hormones play a significant role in how you feel after childbirth.

Baby blues only last a few weeks because they directly result from fluctuating hormone levels, which tend to even out a few weeks after giving birth (Schiedel, 2023). You will get a rush of oxytocin to bond with your baby, which impacts the mother-bear aspect in many new parents. While this feeling can help you feel protective of your baby, it can also increase your anxiety as you navigate being responsible for this helpless little creature in such a big, bad world.

A less discussed hormonal issue is postpartum thyroiditis or inflammation of your thyroid gland. There is no distinct cause, but the symptoms closely resemble postpartum depression, including anxiety, insomnia, irritability, fatigue, weight gain, and depression (Schiedel, 2023). Remember to always reach out to your care provider to let them know what is going on so we can help address these.

How Prolactin Affects Your Menstrual Cycle

Prolactin helps with breast tissue and milk production, which can interrupt your menstrual cycle. When your newborn suckles during breastfeeding, they promote more prolactin production. This is why many women lack regular menstrual cycles while breastfeeding. Some women will get their menses back even with exclusive nursing. I happened to be one of those women, and wow, I was annoyed! What a rip-off! If you are lucky enough to be one who does not get their periods back while nursing, just be aware that you can get pregnant! You can ovulate before you have a period, so keep that in mind as you choose to become sexually active again.

If you do not breastfeed, your prolactin levels even out about two weeks after childbirth (Davis, 2023). Your period will most likely come back six to eight weeks after giving birth if you are not breastfeeding; otherwise, it might not come back until you wean your baby (Schiedel, 2023). Your first few periods after giving birth may be irregular.

You should know that breastfeeding moms can have more difficulty with sex. You may struggle with getting self-lubricated and sometimes have a more challenging time being able to orgasm. It can feel as dry as the desert sometimes, which can lead to painful intercourse. This can all turn into a spiral effect of problems if not addressed.

Postpartum Adrenal Fatigue

Adrenal fatigue can present in sleeping issues, craving junk food, relying on caffeine to wake up, and feelings of overall exhaustion (Davis, 2023). Again, it can feel difficult to discern between new parenthood, postpartum mood disorders, and postpartum adrenal fatigue since there is so much overlap.

This is a tricky topic to discuss when patients specifically ask about it. It is not an official diagnosis but rather a complex interplay of many systems that can significantly get out of whack postpartum. It is an all-encompassing "label" (Mishra, 2022).

After childbirth, your body can produce unreliable levels of steroid hormones and epinephrine, so you should consult your provider for more information on hormonal balance if you experience these symptoms. There are adrenal hormone supplements that can give you a necessary boost, but it is unhealthy to take them if you do not need them, so get professional approval first.

For example, there are no official tests or labs to do assessments for this. Sure, there are adrenal tests that can be taken, and they are important to rule out some other medical complications, but not in the same way that we can test for diabetes, for example. This is still more talked about in the alternative medicine world, which needs to be discussed. It can be difficult to explain well without discounting it, so talk to a medical provider you trust for more information.

What to Do to Support the Rebalancing of Your Hormones

Your hormones will continue to fluctuate naturally after giving birth. Can I start by saying I *hate* it when people try to sell you on "balancing your hormones"? There are no magic recipes to do this. No perfect lab draw will tell us precisely what you need as far as hormones go. This is especially true in the world of perimenopause/menopause. Your brand-new nursing mom's hormones can differ significantly from a six-month postpartum mama. However, taking care of yourself is one of the best ways to help your body find its homeostasis of hormones. Think of the three S's to help with hormone regulation: sleep, safety, and satiety. These three concepts can help with many aspects of your life, including big hormone changes. You should get as much rest as possible, giving your body downtime to level everything out. Sleep will also boost cortisol production so you can stay calm and anxiety-free.

Eating well can also help your hormones regulate naturally. Added benefits of a balanced diet include overall better health, an increase in energy levels, better sleep hygiene, and the ability to manage your weight and exercise easily (Davis, 2023).

THE POWER OF BODY ACCEPTANCE

Loving your new body may feel nearly impossible if you hardly recognize yourself or feel uncomfortable, but you do not need to force body positivity on yourself. You can aim for body neutrality for a beneficial outcome—instead of loving or hating your body. You accept it as it is, a powerful machine keeping you and your newborn alive and thriving!

When you experience a negative body thought, reframe it. Again, you do not have to turn it into a glowing review of your beauty—neutralize it. Ignore how your body looks in the mirror, but focus on what it does for you and your baby. The number on the scale does not matter, and you do not need to try to fit back into your pre-pregnancy clothes. Even if you lose all the baby weight, your body shape may change, so those clothes do not mean anything anymore.

Embrace Your New Body

You can embrace your new body by being kind and compassionate, accepting this as they are without pushing yourself to physical exhaustion. Body positivity is a good goal, but the movement has its fair share of issues. For example, body positivity focuses on the appearance of bodies, which does not matter in the long run. It is more important to focus on what your body is capable of, especially when you are a new mom marveling over pregnancy, childbirth, and the ability to get through every day.

However, the general mindset behind body positivity—of loving your physical self and embracing it as it is now without putting too much energy and negativity into changing it, is crucial during the postpartum period. It may feel challenging to identify yourself in your current body after going through so many changes. You may have struggled with stretchmarks and changing shapes and weight in unexpected places. However, even if you do not look like your ideal, you should accept your body and appreciate how it got you to this point of motherhood, fostering your baby's growth, birth, and continuing help.

One key to body positivity is to dress in a way that feels comfortable. Do not feel like you cannot pull off a particular style because of your body shape or because you are a mother now. Dress in a comfortable, enjoyable way that makes you feel good. You might find it easiest to wear simple styles so you feel put together without spending an hour trying different clothes each morning. Find what you like and buy the same item in different colors or patterns for a go-to "mom uniform" that makes you feel good and comfortable without much thought or stress. Everyone has that one top or outfit that makes them feel like a rock star! You smile at yourself when you see it in the mirror! Find that new outfit! Find that top that makes you spin, and take a long look at how cute you are!

Many moms worry about stretch marks, trying to find that miracle serum that completely erases them. About 50% of women get stretch marks as adults, typically after pregnancy, though weight gain and loss can cause these lines (Matrescence Skin, 2023). It is easy to think these marks are ugly or undesirable because all you see on social media, TV, and magazines are perfect skin. Spoiler alert: It is all airbrushed! It is fake! Skin does not look like that, even for women who never had a baby. Stretch marks are not something you should try to erase but rather wear like a badge of honor. They show how your body grew to accommodate a human, which is incredible! These stretch marks are an important part of your story, and embracing them empowers you to love your body completely. Sometimes our little nuggets leave us little souvenirs. And it is nothing you did or did not do. Contrary to some companies' marketing, no magic cream or lotion can prevent stretch marks. Blame it on genetics! There are so many things we cannot control, and this happens to be one of them.

When you feel good about how you look and what you wear, positive self-talk can come more naturally. You will feel free enough to focus on important daily tasks instead of worrying about how your body looks because you know what it is capable of doing.

Build Body Confidence

No matter what you feel about your body, it is justified, and you should allow yourself to feel it. However, adjusting your expectations so you are not pushing yourself to be super-model thin a week after having a baby is important. In fact, stop relying on the mirror and scale to tell you about your body and let yourself feel whatever you need to feel. Stay off social media and its unrealistic expectations and go with the flow.

Building body confidence comes from within—you should love yourself inside and out, and then you will realize that nothing else matters. I know this can seem unrealistic and overwhelming. But if you prioritize self-care, giving yourself time to get back in touch with your body after it has done such an amazing thing as giving birth, you will understand how powerful your body is, learn how to treat it well, and value all it has done for you.

Once you give birth, there is no baby inside you, so you have already lost weight, right? Technically accurate, but think of how much your body changed to accommodate the baby. Your blood volume increased, and you had a placenta, amniotic fluid, and more. Not just a baby! You produce relaxin to allow your joints to become more flexible for the baby's growth and birth. Your feet and hips may have spread and stay that way. You might be the same size as before, but your jeans do not fit the same because your body shape changes in more ways than just gaining weight. It can be hard to accept these changes that impact your body more than gaining weight alone.

There is no need to stick to a postpartum diet if the focus is losing weight—staying healthy and eating a balanced diet is most important right now. Prioritize exercise that energizes you and makes you feel good instead of what burns the most calories. Finding the right routine of healthy meals, moderate exercise, and clothes that make you feel comfortable can help you build body confidence when it can significantly impact your mental and emotional health.

POSTPARTUM MUST-HAVE ITEMS

Instead of thinking about magical serums to erase stretch marks and how you cannot fit into your pre-pregnancy clothes, use the fourth trimester to focus on self-care by using these must-have postpartum items to help you feel your best and promote healing. Fair warning: These items are far from glamorous, but they will make you feel so comfortable and cared for that you should not deny yourself.

- **Maternity robe:** comfortable, cozy, and easy to wear for breastfeeding
- **Postpartum belly band:** supports your abdomen while you heal
- **Tucks pads:** Witch hazel pads to relieve pain and inflammation
- **Dermaplast:** spray to alleviate pain and itching
- **Epsom salt:** Add to a sitz bath to alleviate pain and take time to relax
- **Adult diapers:** protection, just in case!
- **Mesh underwear:** Prevent staining your regular underwear and have room for pads

- **Postpartum care pads:** infused with natural ingredients to promote healing
- **Peri-bottle:** Easily wash your perineum after using the bathroom
- **Perineal cold packs:** Apply cold to your perineum to alleviate pain
- **Body wipes:** Stay clean without needing a shower
- **Prenatal vitamin:** Boost your nutrition while you heal and breastfeed

If you are breastfeeding, keep these self-care items on hand:

- **Heat and ice pack:** Heat can increase breast milk flow, and ice can relieve pain
- **Manual silicone breast pump:** store your milk, promote latching, and catch leaks
- **Nursing bras:** soft yet supportive and easy to use on-demand
- **Cooling pads:** Gel pads relieve nipple pain between feedings
- **Nipple butter:** Soothe yourself by preventing cracked and bleeding nipples
- **Nipple pads:** prevent leaks staining your clothes

If you are not breastfeeding, you want to find a supportive sports bra or Ace bandage wrap paired with ice packs.

These items can feel like necessities, but they are also a great way to prioritize self-care as you give yourself the time and grace to heal after giving birth.

INTERACTIVE ELEMENT

This chapter's goal is to empower you to accept and love your body as it is because you just went through some major changes. The tips in the previous sections should help you adjust your expectations in the fourth trimester, empowering you to embrace body positivity. These affirmations can also help you create and foster an environment of self-love and body acceptance.

- My body is strong and unique.
- My body created this tiny, wonderful human.
- I am grateful that my body created this miracle.
- My body is enough to sustain me.
- It does not matter how my body looks because I know the strength it contains.
- My body has shown me that it is stronger than I ever thought possible.
- I am proud of everything my body can do.
- My body is helping me do everything I need to do as a new mom, and I love it for that reason.
- I accept that my body looks different because it just created a baby.
- My body is healing and will continue to heal because it is amazingly self-sufficient.
- I am worthy of sleep, safety, and satiety.

KEY TAKEAWAYS

Your body changes during pregnancy and after childbirth for many reasons, with hormones being a significant factor. Hormones will also impact your mood and sense of well-being.

- Giving birth is not the end of many physical changes, as you will still experience discharge, engorgement, and other discomfort relating to the end of pregnancy.
- Hormones can impact your mental health as well as your physical body, so stay aware of how they can cause baby blues and change your menstrual cycle.
- Body acceptance is crucial for new moms because you should embrace all this amazing physical vessel has done for you and your baby! However, it can take time to reach that place. Finding ways to neutralize your relationship with your body can help your mental and emotional health, so follow the steps in the previous sections to embrace where you are right now.

After spending time focusing on your body and self-love, why not turn that acceptance outward and see how your new mom identity connects with your partner and social circle? Read on to learn how to initiate quality communication and set boundaries with people in your life.

I would love to hear from you!

Do you know someone that this book could help? Its by your support and reviews that my book is able to reach other pregnant and postpartum families. Please take 60 seconds to kindly leave a review on Amazon. Please scan the QR code below. If you are in a country that isn't listed, please use the link provided by your Amazon order.

Please follow these steps to rate and review my book

- Open your camera on your phone
- Hover over the QR code
- Rate/Review my book

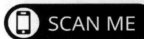
SCAN ME

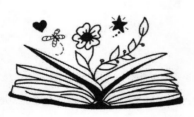

5

GET TO KNOW THE NEW MOM IN YOU—CULTIVATING CONNECTIONS WITH SELF, PARTNER, AND OTHERS

A loving relationship is one in which the loved one is free to be himself—to laugh with me, but never at me; to cry with me, but never because of me; to love life, to love himself, to love being loved.

— LEO BUSCAGLIA

It may feel tough to be your true self after becoming a mother. You are juggling a new identity that can completely consume your life, but it is possible to integrate this new role with the rest of yourself to become a new version of your best self. As you adapt to the change personally, you will feel better prepared to cultivate stronger connections with your partners and others, which will help you feel supported and make it easier to adjust to the major life change of becoming a parent.

REDISCOVERING YOURSELF

There is a balance to rediscovering yourself while embracing your new mother role. You can still be the same person you were before pregnancy with new, exciting additions. For example, you can still take your morning walk, but now you can bring your baby. You can also change your routine, adding visits to a children's museum to provide enrichment for your child while still enjoying your life. Adding new things to your routine can help you feel invigorated so you do not feel bogged down in the basic ways of new motherhood.

One key factor to rediscovering yourself is to allow a grieving period for your previous life. Things will never be the same, and once you are sleeping in five-minute bursts and wearing clothes with spit-up crusted on the shoulder, you will naturally grieve for what you had. You should not feel guilty for feeling this way—it is normal to miss certain phases of your life, and it does not mean you regret having your baby or want to return to how you lived before giving birth. It is just different, so you must allow yourself the time to adapt to that change. The new you is pretty great too!

Understanding your expectations will also impact your feelings about yourself and your new life. Society and social media make it seem like every new mother will immediately embrace motherhood and become this beautiful, peaceful creature that can do it all. That is not reality, so do not expect that of yourself. You can acknowledge that you will not be the person you were a year ago, but you should also outline your expectations. What hobbies do you want to bring back into your postpartum life? How can you ensure there is time for these hobbies? What can you do to make this time for yourself? Do not feel like you need to give up sleep to make it happen—think logically about your priorities to give your most important needs the time and attention they deserve.

It is natural to feel like you are losing yourself since a baby's needs always seem to come first. You may have lost control over your schedule and how you spend your time because you are basically at your baby's beck and call. In addition to that disruption, you are still healing from pregnancy and birth, and your body may feel completely foreign. You do not feel like yourself mentally or physically, and overcoming how swiftly this disruption took over your life can be hard. It can make you feel anxious and stagnant at the same time.

While many people love being a mother, it is also natural not to feel like a born caregiver. You can be a good mother without feeling like it was your sole purpose on Earth. In fact, you may feel more like yourself if you do not define yourself as a mother. That term can feel limiting to many people and make them feel like they should be doing more for their baby instead of focusing on redefining themselves and feeling true to themselves.

Give yourself time alone each day, even if it is just a few minutes when you wake up or before sleep. Do not try to accomplish anything concrete during this time—spend time with yourself and your thoughts. If you can find more time for yourself, like enjoying coffee or tea alone while the drink is still hot, then prioritize those moments. You will feel more in tune with yourself and can better care for others since you know you will always get a few moments alone.

It would help if you got out of the house to feel like yourself. It can feel stifling and isolating to stay home with your baby all the time, so going for a drive may help. If possible, go alone or to the grocery store once a week—something to get out of the house. If you need to bring your baby, consider trying to find a playgroup or mommy and me music or yoga class. You will leave the house, bond with your baby, and meet other parents. You do not have to drive, either—going for a walk or sitting in a coffee shop can be enough of a change of scenery that you feel more in touch with yourself just from this bit of time alone.

Setting goals for yourself can also help you get back in touch with yourself and understand how you want to move forward. It enables you to focus on something other than motherhood, though your goals can still relate to your role as a mother or your child's well-being. However, this is your time to dream. Write goals about wanting to prioritize your creative hobby, reading a book every month, or getting that promotion when you go back to work. Your family can absolutely be part of your goals, but you still want to prioritize yourself.

ENCOURAGING OPEN COMMUNICATION WITH YOUR PARTNER

When navigating new parenthood, you may have so much on your plate that communicating with your partner takes a backseat to everything else, like getting through the day with little to no sleep. You might think your partner can figure out what to do and how to support you. However, keeping open lines of communication can make a big difference in your daily life and parenting journey.

Both you and your partner are adjusting to parenthood, so remember that you are both working with stress and sleep deprivation. With that in mind, it is best to talk about things openly when you both feel rested enough to have a conversation without feeling attacked or cranky. Give each other grace so if you do snap at each other, you can let it go, acknowledging that it is the state of things, not a true reflection of how you feel about each other (Fletcher, 2016).

While you want to spend time alone to get back in touch with your true self and understand how you have changed and who you want to be moving forward, your partner is also part of this equation. Spending time with them during the fourth trimester can strengthen your bonds in many ways. You can be together as a family to understand your dynamics better, but you should also spend time alone with your partner while the baby sleeps or on a date while a trusted friend or family member babysits.

You can do things together to lighten each person's work-load while spending time bonding. For example, maybe you make meals together or go on a morning walk together. You can start watching a new show together and bond over what you like best or think will happen in the next episode. Sometimes focusing on something other than the baby and your new roles as parents can help you stay true to each other and relieve some of the pressure you feel as a caregiver.

How to Share Parenting Responsibilities

We have established that the United States sucks for post-partum care, so it is entirely possible that your partner cannot be home with you after you have the baby. However, if your partner has parental leave from work, they should strongly consider taking it. They can take it right after the baby is born to give you time to heal while you all bond as a family. Maybe they take it when your leave is up so someone can stay home with the baby while the other works. If you have this leave available, consider how to schedule it to benefit the entire family and share parenting responsibilities in any way possible.

New mothers often feel like they are carrying the bulk of the load since they are healing from birth and often take on much of the baby's primary care (Philpott, n.d.). However, talking openly with your partner about the responsibilities is crucial. It can be common for some women to feel resentful of their partner at times. Their body did not change, and they did not need time to heal. Their life may not have had the massive change that yours did. So, you need to talk about it! It can feel tough to ask your partner to take on parenting responsibilities if they are still working while you stay home with the baby, but sharing the load at this stage is crucial. You need to heal, and they need to understand that they are an equal parent. You both will need to help carry the load, but it is not demanding to ask your partner to pick up more of the slack during the fourth trimester when your body needs to heal and your emotions need to regulate. Trade-off certain tasks and take shifts to allow each of you a chance at a full night's sleep. While ensuring that you both help take care of the house, prioritize spending equal time bonding with the baby and having quiet time.

I also think it is just fine to write a "chore list". Making an obvious list and putting it on the fridge can help solidify new routines. The list does not always need to be there, but while there is a time of major change in your life, having something in writing can help organize tasks in the long run.

Perhaps your partner is not aware of how many times the bottles need to be cleaned initially. Or what the day-to-day tasks of the household look like. Writing it up may be easier to decide who will do what. You can also set up a weekly meeting to go over who can do what. It's a great time to check in with each other and you can bring up things that perhaps were put on the backburner to discuss.

Along with its many flaws, the United States seems to infantilize partners, especially fathers. They are not treated like true parents because society applauds them for doing the bare minimum. They "babysit" their kids when the mother goes out instead of just being the parent. So, it is important for you to speak up if you find yourself in this position with your partner. They need to carry an equal load of parenthood. Our cultural norms have been changing and what the family roles were in 1972 are not that of our current families.

I also want to add something about moms' "gatekeeping." There is more than one way to change a diaper, rock a baby, or pick what outfit they can wear. Let your partner figure it out. While it may be tempting to "do it the right way" or take over because it is easier to do it yourself, that does not help in the long run. Having a few different ways to do the same thing is just fine.

Showing Gratitude to Your Partner

It can feel easy to keep track of points at this time—you breastfeed and pump, so you are doing X and Y, while your partner is still working a full-time job and grocery shopping, so what is that worth to you? This type of thinking is detrimental—you should remember that you are a team, both working toward the same goal. When you let go of keeping track of who did what, you will appreciate your partner's contributions more and not feel bitterness over what you are doing compared to what they are doing.

It is ideal to share your strengths and weaknesses when sharing parenting duties. If you love cooking, you can handle meals while your partner washes and cleans the kitchen. They could handle lawn care, and you clean the bathrooms. You can show gratitude by doing your work and appreciating that they are doing something you do not want to or cannot handle, especially as you heal. Acknowledging what your partner is doing can also change the dynamics of working through times that you both may feel exhausted. "I know you're really tired too, but you still finished all the dishes and put them away." In turn, they may start to see all the invisible work that you are doing too.

You can also show gratitude by being kind when communicating with your partner. One great way to do this is to use "I" statements instead of having your words come out like you are starting an argument. For example, instead of saying, "You always let me get up in the middle of the night instead of giving the baby a bottle," you can say, "I feel like I am losing sleep because I always get up in the night, even though I made bottles. Could you take over a few feedings using the bottles?" When you tell your partner how you feel instead of accusing them, they will understand the impact of their actions (or lack thereof) and know how they can step up to help. It is always easier to hear a statement of acknowledgement and needs instead of accusatory or attacking.

Creating a United Front in Parenting

You want to create a united front in parenting, giving you and your partner a strong sense of teamwork as your child grows up. When you are a united front, you know what each of you expects from your child. You know how to approach parenting in a way to raise a person you are both proud of and who represents the best of you both.

You probably talked extensively about parenting before you decided to have a baby and during the pregnancy. You both know the type of parents you want to be, though this ideal can shift when you bring the baby home. Talking through these expectations, changes, and realities can help establish a united front.

Even if you talked about your parenting styles before having a baby, you must accept that you are different people and will react differently. Remember that you were raised differently, so your sense of "normal parenting" may differ. Your partner may have a more playful approach with bath time while you just want to get it done so you and the baby can sleep. When it is your partner's time to bathe the baby, take that opportunity to do your own thing. Do not stay close by and micromanage how they bathe the baby because it is their responsibility and bonding time, so you should take that time to be with yourself, resting or relaxing.

To build a foundation for a united parenting front, you should strive to keep open lines of communication. You will want to find ways to bring up problems neutrally, so no one feels attacked. As mentioned above, using "I" statements is a great way to do this. You should each have a chance to talk and feel heard, suggesting solutions for the problem without interruption. You should both agree on the solution and how to implement it. Being your own biggest advocate with what your needs are can help prevent buildup of resentment. You have the power to self-promote more than anyone.

Intimacy With Your Partner

As you juggle parenthood, intimacy may be the last thing on your mind, especially as you heal from a vaginal birth or C-section. As mentioned in Chapter 4, your changing hormones also impact your ability to self-lubricate or orgasm from sex, making you wonder, *what is the point?*

Your provider will recommend waiting at least six weeks after giving birth before engaging in sex, giving your body enough time to heal from tears, episiotomies, or C-section incisions. However, that does not mean you must be ready to go when you reach that benchmark. Six weeks was a benchmark that many providers would use because that is when pregnancy "care" typically ended. This time frame is not for everyone! You are the decision maker as to when you are ready.

If you have sex a few weeks after giving birth, consider using lubricant to alleviate vaginal dryness. Be careful regarding protection if you are not ready to get pregnant again. Even if you do not get your period due to breastfeeding, you can still get pregnant. You will ovulate the month before your period returns, so it is better to be careful while juggling new parenthood and your newborn. Providers often recommend waiting 18 to 24 months between pregnancies if possible, so you will want to prioritize protection (Mayo Clinic, n.d.-a).

A little over-the-counter lube can go a long way! Just the basic stuff is fine. Water-based or silicone-based is fine. Be aware that oil can break down latex condoms, so be careful using coconut oil for lubrication. Painful sex due to vaginal dryness is a great way to set up a cascade of problems. No one wants to do something that hurts! And if it does hurt, it will trigger your brain to be worried or fearful for future sexual encounters. A woman's main sex organ is the brain! And that needs the most love and care of all!

Be upfront about your desires and expectations. If you are not ready for vaginal sex, tell your partner. There are many other ways to experience intimacy, like holding hands, kissing, massaging each other, oral sex, or mutual masturbation.

You can still feel physically close to your partner without having sex.

Helpful Things to Do and Say

This section is for your partner to read. Go ahead, and hand the book to them. I'll wait.

Hello, partner! This section will help you understand how you can support your loved one as they adjust to motherhood and heal after giving birth. Society hides many aspects of the fourth trimester, making it seem like new mothers should bounce back to "normal" after having a baby, but that is simply not the case. The things on this list can help you support your partner in many ways, including strengthening your relationship with them and your bond with your newborn. Remember, this is not 1952, so keep an open mind and consider applying this advice to your life and partnership to strengthen your growing family.

- **Be patient.** Your partner just underwent a major life change, from pregnancy to childbirth. The changes to their body alone are astronomical! They may never return completely to their previous self because they are adjusting to parenthood and all their physical, mental, and emotional changes.
- **Encourage your partner to talk about their feelings.** They will feel supported even if you listen and do not offer advice. Truly listen to them and try to think of ways to support them without asking

them what you should do. For example, if they experience insomnia, offer to take night shifts for a few nights instead of leaving it to your partner to ask you. Active listening is so important. This does not mean you need to "fix something" necessarily. Sometimes new moms just need to be heard and validated. Asking your partner if they want to talk it out and are looking for validation or if they are looking for advice is important. This can carry on beyond postpartum. It is a great thing to ask in many aspects of your partnership.

- **Care for the baby when you can.** Even if you are working while your partner stays home, they do not need to be with the baby 24/7. They need time alone or away from the house. Take the baby on a walk so your partner can sleep. Perhaps encourage them to go out for coffee with a friend while you handle the baby's nighttime routine. The Pew Research Center found that even when hetero partners earn the same, women still do more housework and caregiving (Chavda, 2023). The *only* time domestic work is split 50/50 is when the male partner does not work at all. Let that sink in a bit. Maybe this next generation can look at "partnerships" and what that really means. My point is that you most likely can do more.

- **Suggest spending time together.** Cook together, watch movies together, and go on walks together. You are making the plan, and inviting your partner along makes it more likely they will relax and say yes because all they have to do is go with the flow instead of organizing everything themselves.

- **Be accountable.** Nothing is worse than someone saying they will do something and not do it. Trust issues and resentment can be tough for relationships to come back from, so do not even make it an issue from the start of this new journey together. Additionally, if you say you will do something, do it and close the loop. As in finishing the task completely. If you are "going to do the dishes," do them all—including putting them away. Leaving tasks halfway finished is not really doing the full task.

Above all, talk with your partner about what others can do to help. Remember, it is not the two of you against the world —you have a support network of people who can help. Who can watch the baby for a date night? Can you order groceries for the week? Hire a cleaner and landscaping crew for a few months to free up time?

But also, be careful to ask your partner to "tell you what they need." This can increase many mothers' mental load, and asking them to give you that information can worsen it. There are ways to ask them without making it harder for them.

Weaponized incompetence is when you pretend you cannot complete a household task or say that the mother does it better, meaning that you will not help at all, leaving the work for the mother (Abramson, 2022). You may sloppily fold laundry, making it so wrinkled that the mother needs to rewash it and fold it herself in frustration. The task was done correctly, but the main issue is that the mother still did it all, not you. You are not carrying the load and helping out.

This can become a major issue for new parents, especially if the mother breastfeeds. You may feel like you cannot help with feeding at all. If the mother pumps a bottle, you may act like you do not know when the baby is hungry, when they are full, or how to burp them.

If your partner starts picking up your slack, you will feel rewarded for your weaponized incompetence and may start using it even more, even if that is not your intention. The mother will be doing the vast majority of the parenting and household tasks at a time when she needs to prioritize self-care and healing. Besides feeling put upon in that way, she may also start to resent you and stop trusting you. After all, you do not know how to do some household chores—what else might you pretend you do not know how to do? It is a slippery slope that can tax her mentally at a time she should be taking it easy.

It will be harder to stop using this tactic when you start getting away with weaponized incompetence. Talk to your partner about the workload and what you should take on because they need to heal. Try to figure out why you are acting like that. Be willing to compromise with issues, like handling tasks your partner does not like. You can also compromise on how tasks should be done, striving less for perfection and more for completion, at least during this phase of your life.

This may not be you at all, and if that is the case, great! However, our statistics in this country show otherwise. Remember, our culture was made to benefit the patriarch, not an equal partnership. So, just read this with an open mind.

Now you can hand this book back to your partner. They need to read this next section while you get to work cooking or cleaning or doing laundry or…

UNDERSTANDING THE IMPORTANCE OF HELP FROM OTHERS

Society makes mothers feel like they can and should do it all, but that is not reality. Help from others makes more of an impact than you can believe. Whenever possible, outsourcing, delegating, and automating tasks will make a huge difference in your workload. You can then give yourself the time and space to be with your baby or spend time alone, relaxing, or getting back in touch with some of your favorite hobbies from before you had a baby.

People want to help! Sometimes taking on the mental load of delegating can be exhausting in and of itself. As silly as it may sound, list five easy things you can have someone do for you when they ask. Put the list on the fridge so people can see it, or you can quickly glance at it when they visit or call.

Some ways of delegating and outsourcing include asking friends to pick up certain grocery store items during their own shopping trips. These days you can also use services like Instacart or grocery delivery to simplify the task of stocking your kitchen. You can hire someone to walk your dog, mow the lawn, or clean the house. You can have a meal delivery subscription to simplify meal planning. Remember that you do not have to commit to these services forever—just for a few weeks or months to give yourself the time to heal and adjust to life without feeling overwhelmed and outsourcing for the win!

SETTING BOUNDARIES

Not all advice is good advice, so setting boundaries is crucial, especially as a new parent. You want to feel in control when people come to your house or give you unsolicited advice. Thinking about boundaries before you find yourself in an uncomfortable situation empowers you to have a response ready when someone oversteps.

You may have already experienced needing to set boundaries even before the baby was out! Many patients ask about visitor policies where I work because of the number of people wanting to come to the birth that they do not want to be there. Labor and delivery nurses will even set up a safe word with their patients as a cue to get people out of the delivery room! If they ask you if you are ready for your "pineapple juice," and you say yes, they can help clear out the room.

This can be one of the first "parenting" decisions you may need to make. Uncle Hank can wait a few weeks to see the baby instead of the next day at the hospital. Blame it on me!

• "We appreciate your thoughts and well wishes as we welcome our bundle of joy, but we need time together as a family. We will let you know when we are ready for visitors."

• "We are going to schedule a 'meet the baby' gathering as soon as we feel up to it. We will give you more information then."

• "We need time to get to know our little one before inviting people over, so we would prefer not to have visitors at this time."

• "If you plan on stopping by, I need you to check with me first."

Replying to Unsolicited Advice

People want to give new parents advice about everything, from breastfeeding and weaning to sleep routines and immunizations. It does not matter if these advice-givers have children of their own or not—they have opinions, and they are going to share them with you.

It can feel awkward to react to someone giving you unwanted advice. You might feel more comfortable smiling and nodding or dismissing them with a polite "Thank you." However, if you want a statement ready to prevent future advice, you can try some statements like the following:

• "Thank you for your advice, but we are listening to our providers and following their suggestions."

• "Thank you for your advice, but at this point, I need someone to listen more than give feedback."

• "Your advice makes me feel like you are eager to help. More than advice, I would prefer an extra set of hands. Would you mind helping with ___?"

Addressing Too Much Help

While it may seem more beneficial to ask for hands-on help than advice, there can come a time when someone wants to give you too much help or overstays their welcome. Again, this can be an awkward situation, but if you nip it in the bud, it should be clear to the helper exactly what you need and how to prevent this issue in the future. You may want to say something like:

• "We appreciate your help but need some time together as a family right now."

- "Thank you for all you have done! We do not need any help right now, but I will let you know how you can help in the future."
- "We are happy you want to visit, but we need time to find our routine as a new family. Maybe you can stay for X days and book a hotel so we will still have the chance to bond with our newborn while you are in town."
- "What would be helpful to me is if you could handle X, Y, and Z instead of just holding the baby. I am still meeting this little person myself and could use this time to bond."

INTERACTIVE ELEMENT

Many of the interactive elements to this point have helped you work through issues independently, so this is a twist on that concept. A relationship check-in journal gives you and your partner thoughtful time together to track growth in your relationship and with yourselves independently.

*You can write letters to each other, sharing your thoughts about what has happened recently.

*Update the journal at the end of each day, writing down a few notes about the hard tasks you overcame together.

*Share a compliment with your partner, highlighting how they made you feel supported or loved.

*Look ahead to the future. List things you look forward to doing as a family or as a couple with someone watching your baby.

*Take time to share some of your favorite memories, each writing about something from your past that reminds you of the strength of your love.

*Write about memories from your childhoods, which helps you get a complete picture of your partner and how you can work together to provide a loving childhood for your newborn.

KEY TAKEAWAYS

While so much of the fourth trimester is about a mother's healing, it is also important to look at your relationships. Strengthening your partnership and how you feel about your family, friends, and social circle can help you feel loved and empowered.

- Before you can give yourself to others, you need time and space to rediscover yourself. Think about some of your biggest passions from pre-pregnancy. How can you prioritize these hobbies and tasks so you feel in touch with your true self while adapting to motherhood?
- Your relationship with your partner can feel stressed as you adapt to a new routine and lifestyle that does

not allow much sleep or relaxation. Keeping open lines of communication will help prevent arguments and ensure you can work together as a team.

- Support can help you take care of some of the tasks on your plate without needing to tax yourself. Delegate and outsource as much as possible to prioritize yourself and your newborn.

- There is such a thing as too much help and unsolicited advice. Develop boundaries so you know when someone is being too overbearing. Have a statement in mind to let them know when you have had enough.

- This type of support and communication can make you feel healthy and balanced. A proper diet will accentuate this state of being even more. Read on for meal planning strategies and nutrition tips to simplify maintaining a healthy diet during your postpartum period.

6

NOURISH, ENERGIZE, THRIVE— POSTPARTUM NUTRITION AND FITNESS GUIDE

The groundwork of all happiness is good health.

— LEIGH HUNT

Many people forget to eat even if they are not parents. They may get caught up in a task, and time flies by before they pause and realize they skipped lunch or dinner. However, when you are a mother, you cannot let this happen. You will feel weak and unhealthy before you know it. However, maintaining a regular meal schedule can feel insurmountable for new parents. Your focus is your baby: feeding, cleaning, sleeping. It can seem nearly impossible to also provide for yourself. You may exist on granola bars and frozen meals for several weeks after having a baby. However, meal prep is one way to ensure you get quality nutrition when you cannot focus on much more than your healing body and your newborn.

THE ROLE OF PROPER NUTRITION IN POSTPARTUM RECOVERY

While I may have some specific supplements listed below, please know that the FDA does not regulate these. Getting it from your food is ideal, but if you choose supplements, be aware that you may not get what the label implies. Food-based is where it's at!

Proper nutrition aids in postpartum recovery by giving you the fuel your body needs to make it through the day—while also healing itself from pregnancy and childbirth. If you are breastfeeding, your baby gets these nutritious benefits, too. A healthy diet can increase the speed of your recovery. Hydrating well, eating complex carbs, fruits and vegetables, healthy fats, and plenty of protein can help reduce bone loss, prevent hemorrhoids, and replenish your iron stores.

Society makes you feel like you are supposed to strive to get your body back after having a baby, but the true message should be that postpartum wellness is your ultimate priority. This has nothing to do with weight loss or your body shape. Focus on what you put into your body to help it heal versus focusing on what society thinks you should look like.

A balanced diet helps your body heal from pregnancy and childbirth and encourages mental wellness. When your body feels good and you have the energy and nutrients to provide for your baby, you will feel more positive about being a new parent.

Eating warm foods postpartum increases digestion, so soups and stews are quick and easy meals that will provide the comfort and nutrition you need. Balance the warmth with fruits and vegetables, healthy fats, and proteins to promote anti-inflammatory qualities while getting nutrients.

Collagen will help rebuild tissues, so consider adding a supplement to your diet. It also helps with postpartum hair loss, so you can kill two birds with one stone if that is what you are experiencing. Other supplements, like vitamin D3, omegas, and magnesium, can help with breastmilk production and provide key vitamins you might not get in your food.

Vitamin D3 comes from sunlight and animal-based foods, like eggs, cheese, and fish, though you can also take supplements (Stines, 2023). It helps with bone growth, muscle contractions, and converting sugar into energy. Without enough vitamin D, you can lose bone minerals and experience porous, fragile bones as an adult. If your muscles feel weak or you have bone pain, talk to your provider about your D3 levels.

Omega-3s are a group of essential fatty acids that have numerous health benefits. Your body does not naturally make enough omegas, so you should get them from your diet. These can include fatty fish like salmon, sardines, flaxseed, and chia seeds. Getting enough omega-3 improves heart health, reduces the risk of cardiovascular disease, and can protect against Alzheimer's, dementia, and some forms of cancer, including breast cancer (Cleveland Clinic, 2019).

Magnesium can come in a range of supplements, like citrate, sulfate, glycinate, and more. It can help with the nervous system, muscle function, blood sugar regulation, blood pressure regulation, and making DNA! It can also help with headaches and help you poop! It is found in dark leafy greens, beans, and seeds like pumpkin, hemp, flax, tuna, brown rice, quinoa, almonds, avocados, and dark chocolate (Griffin, 2008).

Choline supports memory and brain health, so you want to add this to your postpartum diet. You can find it in egg yolks, beef, mushrooms, chicken breasts, fish, and potatoes (Chamlou, 2023).

Iron keeps your blood healthy and can greatly affect your energy levels. You may feel dizzy, weak, or tired if you do not have enough iron. You can also have brittle nails, lose your hair, and always feel cold. Women lose blood in childbirth, so talk to your provider about monitoring your iron levels postpartum. You can take a supplement if necessary or eat iron-rich foods like dark leafy greens, beans, lentils, fortified hot cereal, and dark chocolate, to name a few! Organ and red meat, turkey, clams, mussels, and tuna are also high in iron (Chamlou, 2023).

Zinc keeps your immune system functioning at a healthy level, but pregnant and breastfeeding people often have a deficiency. You may notice that your wounds take longer to heal, you lose hair, or you experience postpartum depression and anxiety. You may need a zinc supplement, but you can naturally boost those levels by eating red meat, poultry, oysters, crab, lobster, nuts, and whole grains (Chamlou, 2023).

If you do not eat a balanced diet or skip meals, your hormone levels can fluctuate, greatly impacting your mood and sense of well-being. For example, you will have higher cortisol levels if you skip meals, which can increase your blood pressure and make you irritable due to an influx of stress hormones.

Fiber and hydration also help promote healthy digestion, keeping your "poop" regular. A healthy diet can help keep everything in check for you and your newborn.

THE BENEFITS OF MEAL PREP

Meal prep has many benefits, like eliminating the stress of cooking every meal. You can create meals several days in advance with just a little more time than you would normally need to cook one serving. This lowers the stress of constantly cooking, not to mention the indecisiveness of wondering what you should eat. It is easier to eat every meal when you know something waits in the fridge or freezer instead of feeling the overwhelming dread of cooking something from scratch.

When you prepare meals in advance, you can create something healthy to give you the nutrition you need without needing much mental energy, especially if you feel tired, overwhelmed, or have decision fatigue. Instead of getting so hungry, you eat every snack in the pantry, use the prepared meals to empower yourself to eat a healthy choice, which can lead to weight loss and prevent obesity. You will know you are eating a balanced diet and can prevent yourself from eating unhealthy snacks or getting "hangry" because you went too long without food (Blanton, 2022).

Meal prep is a great way to use everything in your kitchen. You can go to the grocery store (or order your items for delivery!) and immediately prepare them for a week of meals. You will save money because you are eating everything you bought at the store instead of going out to eat or ordering takeout. Meal prepping with your groceries also reduces food waste since you will not forget some lost produce at the back of the fridge and let it spoil before you can eat it.

You will also get emotional benefits from meal prepping. You will always have a warm, fresh meal on hand without needing to stress out and do all the work yourself three times a day, which can help you feel cared for.

Meal Planning Strategies

When you plan meals in advance, you can take time to make healthy choices without feeling overwhelmed by hunger at the moment. You can choose whole foods that fuel your body and provide nutrition for you and your baby. During this postpartum stage, you should focus on eating plenty of protein, fruits and vegetables, fiber-rich carbohydrates, and fats in nuts, seeds, and avocados.

Your nutrition needs may vary depending on your size and activity level, so ensure you eat enough calories to fuel your body. If breastfeeding, you may need to eat up to 2,500 calories daily to encourage milk production (Lindberg, 2020b). You may also need to follow a special diet if you have a health condition like diabetes or Crohn's disease. If you are unsure about the healthiest choices for you, work with your provider to ensure you get enough calories and nutrients for your body.

Hydration is a key part of postpartum health. You should drink at least 128 ounces of water daily to stay hydrated and promote milk production if breastfeeding (White, 2022).

Meal planning does not require you to be a chef. These simple ideas will give you an idea of what you should be eating after giving birth to fuel your body in a healthy way (Lindberg, 2020b).

Breakfast Ideas

- 5 oz. Greek yogurt with a cup of strawberries, topped with a teaspoon of honey and a tablespoon of chia seeds
- Smoothie made with 1½ cups of frozen fruit, 1 cup of protein powder, a cup of spinach or kale, and a cup of almond milk
- 2 eggs scrambled with vegetables with a slice of whole wheat toast
- An egg, half a banana, and a slice of toast topped with ¼ of an avocado

Lunch and Dinner Ideas

- ½ cup of whole wheat pasta with ½ cup of tomato sauce and 3 meatballs
- 4 oz. of chicken or fish with ½ cup of brown rice and 2 cups of vegetables
- 2 tablespoons of peanut butter and a tablespoon of jelly on whole wheat bread
- Two cups of lettuce topped with 2 cups of vegetables and 3 oz. of protein

Snack Ideas

- Protein bars
- 2 tablespoons of hummus with 2 oz. of pita chips

- Carrot and celery sticks
- An apple, string cheese, and a handful of pistachios

Postpartum Nutrition Tips

Avoid diets for weight loss. This is not the time to focus on losing weight because you need to stay as healthy as possible for yourself and your newborn. Extreme diets restrict calories and healthy foods to promote severe weight loss, so they will not help you parent your baby at this point.

You can continue taking prenatal vitamins during your postpartum period. These vitamins deliver key nutrients you need to stay healthy. If you do not want to continue taking vitamins, talk to your provider about natural ways to get those nutrients in your diet.

Avoid empty calories. It is tempting to snack on whatever is handy, but you will fill up on sugar, sodium, and saturated fats, which will not fuel your body the way you need as a new parent.

Drink less caffeine. It may feel necessary to fuel yourself with coffee if you are running on little to no sleep, but you will eventually crash, which can feel even worse. Eating a balanced diet and drinking plenty of water to fuel your body is better, though you can have up to 300 milligrams of caffeine daily (Lindberg, 2020b).

You should also limit your alcohol intake if you are breastfeeding. While a drink or two may help you feel like you can relax, it can show up in your breastmilk. You can drink in moderation and wait two or three hours before breast-feeding to keep your baby safe. While you may not need to "pump and dump," it is always something to consider. Alcohol can also affect your stress levels and sleep hygiene, so moderation is always the best bet for new parents.

SAFE AND EFFECTIVE POSTPARTUM EXERCISES

Many women hesitate to exercise after giving birth because their bodies just went through so much. Like feeling anxious about your first bowel movement after childbirth, the idea of working out can make you worry about causing damage and pain. However, you can do many safe and effective exercises to promote health without harming your postpartum body. Many of these can be done in the comfort of your own home or around your neighborhood. You do not need to join a gym! You can find so many free videos or classes online. However, if you join a gym, use all the facilities. I belonged to a gym that had childcare after my third child. I would work out for 30–45 minutes but still be there for the 2 hours the childcare allowed! The sauna, hot tub, or reading a book in the locker room was always a nice break! And my little (not newborn) loved playing there.

Exercising can strengthen your core, which changes a lot with pregnancy and childbirth. You will also boost your energy levels by exercising, promoting better sleep, relieving stress, and possibly preventing postpartum depression

(Lindberg, 2020a). And while it may seem overwhelming at times to get out there and move your body with a new baby, it is so worth it! It may involve groaning or eye-rolling as you try to talk yourself into getting out there, but no one ever feels worse after they have worked out! Does anyone ever regret exercise? Usually not!

There are four main types of exercise you can do postpartum:

- Aerobic activity
- Moderate intensity
- Vigorous intensity
- Kegel exercises

Aerobic Activity

Aerobic exercises are an excellent way to improve cardiovascular fitness and increase endurance. They involve continuous movement that elevates the heart rate. Postpartum women can engage in low-impact aerobic activities such as walking, swimming, or stationary cycling to minimize stress on joints and muscles. Gradually increasing the duration and intensity of these activities can help mothers regain their pre-pregnancy fitness levels.

Moderate Intensity

Moderate-intensity exercises are essential for postpartum recovery as they help restore muscle tone and strength.

These exercises should focus on the major muscle groups, including the core, arms, legs, and back. Moderate-intensity exercises include bodyweight exercises like squats, lunges, push-ups, and light resistance training with dumbbells or resistance bands. It is crucial to start with lighter weights and gradually increase resistance to avoid injury. I am a huge fan of "bar" type classes. These can be amazing for pelvic floor strength, which will be discussed further.

Vigorous Intensity

Once a new mother has recovered and gained some strength, she can consider incorporating vigorous-intensity activities into her postpartum exercise routine. These exercises are more intense and can further enhance cardiovascular fitness and endurance. Vigorous-intensity exercises include high-intensity interval training (HIIT), kickboxing, or intensive running. Unless you are a professional athlete, I usually do not recommend vigorous exercise until at least 12 weeks postpartum. However, if you are feeling ready for it, go for it! It is important to consult with a healthcare professional before starting vigorous activities to ensure they are suitable for individual recovery progress.

Kegel Exercises

Kegel exercises primarily target the pelvic floor muscles, which can be weakened or strained during pregnancy and childbirth. These exercises involve contracting and relaxing the pelvic floor muscles repeatedly. Kegel exercises can help strengthen the pelvic floor, improve bladder control, and promote postpartum healing. It is recommended to start with a few repetitions of Kegels and gradually increase over time. Consulting with a healthcare professional or a pelvic floor specialist can guide proper technique and progression.

THE BEST POSTPARTUM EXERCISES TO DO NOW

There are some exercises you may be able to do now safely. If you take it easy, you can do these exercises to boost your energy levels and inspire yourself to strive for more activity in your daily life. When you do these exercises and feel ready to move on to something more intense, you can talk to your provider to ensure your body is ready to take that step.

In other countries, they sometimes have a pelvic floor physical therapist evaluate you within the first month. Oh, how I wish this were also the standard of care here! But do know that these amazing people exist! And when we say "physical therapist," know that it is not the same person who may rehab your grandma's broken hip or knee replacement. These are specialists that have additional training specifically for this! It is an entire specialty within the world of PT. There are private practice specialists, and you may need a referral from your provider. Always ask!

Pelvic Floor Exercises

Pelvic floor exercises, known as Kegels, are essential for postpartum recovery. These exercises involve contracting and relaxing the pelvic floor muscles, which can become weakened during pregnancy and childbirth. Kegels help strengthen the pelvic floor, improve bladder control, and aid in the recovery of perineal tissues. Perform Kegels by squeezing the muscles as if stopping the urine flow and holding for a few seconds before releasing. Repeat this exercise several times throughout the day.

Diaphragmatic Breathing

Diaphragmatic breathing is a technique that helps activate the deep core muscles and promote relaxation. To perform this exercise:

- Lie on your back with your knees bent.
- Place one hand on your chest and the other on your belly.
- Inhale deeply through your nose, allowing your belly to rise, and then exhale slowly through your mouth, letting your belly fall.
- Focus on breathing deeply into your diaphragm rather than shallow chest breathing.

Diaphragmatic breathing can help restore abdominal muscle tone and reduce tension.

Walking

Walking is a low-impact exercise that can be easily incorporated into a postpartum routine. It helps improve cardiovascular fitness, promotes circulation, and aids in weight loss. Start with short walks and gradually increase the duration and intensity as you feel comfortable. Walking properly and engaging the core muscles can further enhance the benefits.

Bird Dog Holds

Stability or yoga ball bird dog holds are excellent exercises for strengthening the core, improving balance, and activating the glutes. Start by kneeling on all fours with a ball positioned under your hips. Extend one arm forward and the opposite leg backward while maintaining a stable position on the ball. Hold for a few seconds, engage your core and glutes, and switch sides. This exercise helps restore stability and strength in the postpartum period.

Cat-Cow in Tabletop

Cat-Cow is a gentle yoga movement that promotes spinal mobility and stretches the back muscles. Begin on all fours with your hands under your shoulders and knees under your hips. Inhale as you arch your back, lifting your chest and tailbone toward the ceiling (Cow pose). Exhale as you round your spine, dropping your head and tailbone and tucking your chin toward your chest (Cat pose). Repeat this flow several times, focusing on the movement and stretching sensations.

Stability Ball Glute Bridge

The stability ball glute bridge targets the gluteus muscles, which can become weakened during pregnancy and childbirth. Start by lying on your back with your feet resting on a stability or yoga ball, knees bent, and arms by your sides. Press your feet into the ball as you lift your hips off the ground, forming a straight line from your shoulders to your knees. Squeeze your glutes at the top and then lower your hips back down. This activity helps strengthen the glutes and improve lower body stability.

Modified Planks

Modified planks are an excellent exercise for strengthening the core muscles, including the abdominals, obliques, and back muscles. They also engage the shoulders, arms, and glutes. To perform this plank:

- Position yourself on your forearms and knees with your heels toward the ceiling. This should form a straight line from your head to your knees.
- Engage your core by drawing your belly button toward your spine.
- Hold this position for a set amount of time, starting with 10 to 20 seconds and gradually increasing as you get stronger.
- Focus on maintaining proper form and breathing throughout the exercise. If this is easy and you are

not having discomfort, you can do a full plank on your arms to toes instead of knees.

Side Plank Leg Lifts

Side plank leg lifts are an effective exercise for targeting the obliques, hips, and glutes. This exercise helps strengthen the core and stabilize muscles on the sides of the body. To perform side plank leg lifts, lay on your side with your forearm directly under your shoulder and your legs extended. Lift your hips off the ground, forming a straight line from your head to your heels. Engage your core and lift your top leg while maintaining stability. Lower the leg back down and repeat for several repetitions before switching sides. If the full side plank is too challenging initially, you can modify it by bending the bottom knee and keeping it on the ground for added support.

WHAT YOU DO NOT NEED

It is important to recognize that you do not need to spend excessive money on external forces in your postpartum journey. The health industry often attempts to sell various products like designer pills, meal plans, shakes, and even lactation cookies, promising miraculous results. However, it is crucial to approach these claims cautiously and be aware that many of them are unsupported by scientific evidence.

For example, the market is flooded with pills and meal plans that claim to aid in weight loss, boost energy, or provide specific nutrients for new mothers. While some supplements and dietary modifications may have benefits, consulting with a healthcare professional or a registered dietitian is essential before investing in expensive products. They can provide personalized advice based on individual needs and ensure a balanced and nutritious postpartum diet.

Lactation cookies are often marketed as a solution for new mothers struggling with low milk supply. However, these cookies are not proven to be effective in increasing milk production. While some ingredients like oats and flaxseed may offer nutritional benefits, more than relying on lactation cookies may be misleading and a waste of money. Seeking guidance from a lactation consultant or a healthcare professional is crucial for addressing breastfeeding concerns.

The health industry is driven by profit, and companies may take advantage of vulnerable new mothers by selling products that promise quick fixes or miraculous results. Stay informed and critically evaluate the claims made by these products. Consult reliable sources of information such as healthcare professionals, evidence-based research, and reputable organizations specializing in postpartum care.

Instead of relying solely on expensive external products, new mothers can prioritize holistic approaches to postpartum recovery. This includes engaging in appropriate exercises, maintaining a balanced and nutritious diet, practicing self-care, getting adequate rest, seeking support from healthcare professionals, and building a strong support system.

INTERACTIVE ELEMENT

Creating a postpartum meal plan helps you know what groceries you need and what you should eat at every meal to boost your nutrition, provide enough energy to get through the day, and give your baby what they need through your breast milk.

Healthy diet advice	What I ate
Two servings of whole grains per day (ex: brown rice, farro, quinoa, steel-cut oats)	
Two servings of lean protein per day (ex: chicken breast, turkey, salmon, Greek yogurt, tofu, legumes)	
Two servings of healthy fats per day (ex: nuts, seeds, avocado, fatty fish, chia seeds)	
Plenty of fruits and vegetables	

Postpartum Weekly Meal Plan

Day	Breakfast	Snack	Lunch	Snack	Dinner
Monday					
Tuesday					
Wednesday					
Thursday					
Friday					
Saturday					
Sunday					

KEY TAKEAWAYS

Eating a balanced diet is one of the most important forms of self-care during the postpartum period.

- Meal prep can simplify the work you need to do to eat a healthy meal daily. You, your partner, or a helper can spend a few hours each week preparing meals until your next grocery store delivery or trip.
- Preparing meals in advance ensures you always have healthy food when hungry. You save money by not eating out as much and reduce food waste by purchasing all the groceries.
- When planning meals, ensure a balanced diet with plenty of protein, fruits, and vegetables.
- You may need supplements to get enough of certain vitamins, but eating a balanced diet of whole foods greatly increases the opportunity to get all the nutrients you need.
- Safe exercise will also keep you healthy during the postpartum period. You can do several low-impact exercises without risking the progress your body has made toward healing.
- Do not let the health industry con you: There is no need to buy expensive weight loss pills, tons of supplements or lactation cookies.

7

THE BABY BOND—BEING ONE WITH YOUR BUNDLE OF JOY

Motherhood is a choice you make every day to put someone else's happiness and well-being ahead of your own while not forgetting your own identity.

— DONNA BALL

S ociety makes people think they will immediately fall in love with their baby. I cannot tell you how often I have seen emotional scenes in movies and TV shows where the mother holds her baby for the first time, looks into the baby's eyes, and falls head over heels in love. This can happen, and sure, it is magical. But it could be more realistic. Your body changed drastically over nine to ten months of pregnancy, and you just experienced a human exiting your body. It is understandable if you do not want anyone touching you, much less immediately fall in love with this little crying human who wants still wants to be physically attached to you all the time. You can still be a great mother even if you do not have that experience. And your baby will still be an amazing, well-adjusted person. It takes time to develop a bond with someone, and there is no need to expect bonding with your baby to be any different than getting to know another person.

That said, feeding your baby is a great way to bond. Just as many classic sayings talk about the kitchen being the heart of the home because of all the love and nourishment it provides, you can use this time feeding your baby to bond with them. Whether you breastfeed, bottle feed, or do both, this time is a chance to enjoy quiet with your baby and be with them, developing love.

SKIN-TO-SKIN CONTACT AND BONDING

Skin-to-skin contact typically starts right after birth. This can happen right at delivery and baby can be placed directly on to your chest, and then both of you covered with a warm, dry blanket. This approach calms the baby and can even boost your milk supply. This type of contact promotes better physical and developmental progress for the baby. Regardless of if the baby went to your chest immediately after birth, met you in a recovery room for the first time, or even if it was a few weeks after birth in the setting of a NICU, skin-to-skin will always have benefits!

Why Is Skin-To-Skin Contact Important?

Skin-to-skin contact is important because it helps ground the baby and mother, calming them after the experience of childbirth. When the baby immediately rests on the mother's chest, its heart rate and breathing patterns will regulate to best acclimate it to life outside of the womb. It will also regulate their temperature since they are used to being warm in the womb.

The baby's skin will get the mother's positive bacteria from this contact, helping protect the newborn from infection. The contact also stimulates the release of hormones that help the mother produce breast milk and feel inspired to mother the baby. Similarly, skin-to-skin contact can generate interest in feeding and stimulate digestion in the baby.

Skin-To-Skin Benefits for Babies

Skin-to-skin contact, commonly known as kangaroo care, provides numerous advantages for both the newborn and the adult who perform it.

The ability of newborns to control their body temperature is restricted. Skin-to-skin contact assists the newborn in maintaining a steady body temperature by leveraging the warmth of the caregiver's body. The parent's skin functions as a natural thermostat, altering as needed to keep the infant warm or chilly.

Skin-to-skin contact has been found to aid in the regulation of a baby's heart rate and breathing patterns. It can result in more consistent breathing rates, fewer irregular heartbeat episodes, and better cardiovascular performance (Seitz, 2017).

Early skin-to-skin contact promotes early breastfeeding initiation and a better nursing attachment between the baby and the mother. The baby's innate nursing habits are aided by close physical closeness, which increases the release of hormones that support milk production.

This bonding contact helps the newborn and caregiver form a strong emotional attachment. It instills sentiments of safety, trust, and intimacy. Physical touch causes the production of oxytocin, also known as the "love hormone," which increases feelings of bonding and nurturance.

Skin-to-skin contact provides a soothing touch and proximity that can help relieve tension in both the baby and the caregiver. It has been shown to reduce cortisol levels in newborns, resulting in less crying and improved relaxation (Cleveland Clinic, 2017).

This contact can help preterm and low-birth-weight infants gain weight. Close physical touch aids in the regulation of the baby's metabolism, the conservation of energy, and the promotion of eating (Seitz, 2017).

Skin-to-skin contact exposes the newborn to the mother's natural skin bacteria, which aids in colonizing the baby's microbiome. This exposure can aid in the development of a strong immune system.

Early contact calms newborns, resulting in healthier sleep habits. Close physical contact can help to regulate the baby's sleep-wake cycle, encourage deeper sleep, and enhance overall sleep quality.

According to research, skin-to-skin contact may have long-term benefits for a baby's brain development. It has been linked to greater cognitive performance, stress regulation abilities, and social-emotional development (Unicef, 2023).

MINDFUL PARENTING

Mindful parenting is an approach to parenting that involves being fully present, nonjudgmental, and attentive to the needs of both the parent and the child. It is about cultivating awareness, compassion, and intentional responsiveness in the parent-child relationship. Mindful parenting draws inspiration from the principles of mindfulness, which is the practice of paying attention to the present moment without judgment or reaction. I wish I had known some of these concepts when my kids were little! Even after having four of my own, I see these concepts and think *yes, yes*, and *more yes*!

Mindful parenting is a way to stay present in every aspect of caring for your baby. Instead of letting emotions rule your personality, you let go of any guilt or shame you feel for various reasons and focus on what is happening right now. You will still get angry and upset sometimes, but you will stay level-headed and not let these emotions impact how you interact with your baby. You can acknowledge the feelings without acting on them (Suttie, 2016).

A mindful parent stays aware of their thoughts and feelings without letting emotions rule them—self-regulation as an adult aid in this concept. You act differently when you are calm compared to when you are stressed or angry. Though you will still feel stress and anger, mindful parenting aims to let calm rule over the emotions so you can process them later.

Your goal is to put your child's thoughts, needs, and feelings at the forefront of your mind. You may be operating on little to no sleep, and they keep fussing, so you cannot even eat dinner to give your body some much-needed nutrition and energy. However, you know your baby is fussing for a reason, so you put aside your frustration to stay aware of their needs and act in a responsive manner.

With practice, mindful parenting becomes a way of life. You will find yourself better at regulating your emotions. You will not be critical of yourself or your child because you take everything at face value instead of reading into it. You are less impulsive because you interpret things logically, processing them before you react. As a result, your relationship with your child will improve (Peterson, 2020).

It takes practice to become a mindful parent. Humans are naturally reactive. When someone does something to anger you, most people have the base reaction to retaliate. This might mean you snap at someone who angered you or ignore them because you need to focus on yourself. You cannot do this with your child and still expect to foster a positive relationship, so mindful parenting is a great solution.

If you feel like your emotions will be easily triggered, tell your partner and take a step back. Everyone needs a time out at some point, and it is better to stop yourself before you say or do something you will feel guilty about later. Over time, you will be able to identify your triggers and work to prevent them from becoming an issue as you parent (Suttie, 2016).

Key aspects of mindful parenting include

- **Being present:** The value of being present and engaged with your child is emphasized by mindful parenting. It requires that you pay attention in the current moment, ignore distractions, and actively listen to your child.
- **Nonjudgmental acceptance:** Mindful parenting promotes accepting yourself and your child without judgment. You will let go of preconceived beliefs or expectations and accept your child as they are in the present.

- **Emotional awareness and regulation:** Mindful parenting involves developing emotional awareness in yourself and your child. It promotes emotional recognition and understanding, validates your child's feelings, and teaches appropriate ways of expressing and managing emotions.
- **Empathy and compassion:** Mindful parenting instill empathy and compassion in your child. You will put yourself in your child's shoes, attempting to see their point of view and responding with kindness and understanding.
- **Conscious communication:** Conscious and polite communication with your child is a major factor in mindful parenting. It requires actively listening, communicating with intention and clarity, and constructively expressing your feelings and needs.
- **Self-care and self-compassion:** The need for self-care and self-compassion for the parent is recognized in mindful parenting. It entails looking after yourself, controlling stress, and modeling self-compassion and self-acceptance for your child.
- **Balancing structure and flexibility:** Mindful parenting seeks to create a balance between providing discipline and setting limits, as well as enabling flexibility and adjusting to your child's unique needs and growth (Ceder, 2017).

In the early stages, mindful parenting can be tough because you are adjusting to parenthood and working on little to no sleep. However, starting mindful parenting with a newborn is a great practice to continue as your child gets older, and it will only serve to strengthen your relationship. It is unnecessary to be perfect or always get it right when practicing mindful parenting. It is a never-ending cycle of self-reflection, growth, and learning. You will continually strengthen your connection with your child, reduce stress, and promote a supportive and nurturing atmosphere for their well-being and development by incorporating mindfulness into your parenting style (Peterson, 2020).

Reading to Your Baby

Some people love to relax by reading a book, and others may not read much at all. Either way, you may be surprised to know that you should read to your newborn! Sure, they cannot hold the book or follow along on the page. However, you are giving them crucial language development building blocks that will help them later in life—not only with communication but also in terms of social and emotional development (Gordon, 2022).

A 2019 study found that babies who are read to daily from birth get exposure to about 78,000 words a year (Logan et al., 2019). By age 5, they have heard 1.4 million words, giving them an impressive start to language, reading, and communication.

Reading books with your baby is fun. You are not restricted to the words on the page because your baby is not an impatient listener who wants to know how the story ends. They are happy to hang out with you, so read the text and then talk about the pictures. Point to colors and name them. Identify animals and characters and what they are doing. Talk about what might happen next. You might initially feel silly doing this, but it will give you practice for when you are reading to a very curious toddler who loves to talk about what they see and hear and will establish an amazing bonding routine with your children for years to come.

Babies are born already recognizing their mom's voice. Reading can soothe them, both because you hold them and because they appreciate your voice's tone and rhythm as you read. Try reading for 5 or 10 minutes daily, just a picture book or nursery rhyme during the fourth trimester. You can do it after a bath, bedtime, or nap to help them wake up.

A baby's brain grows so much in their first year of life that they will take in the sounds of language and the images on the page and learn about the meaning of words. Not reading to your baby can be detrimental, with a chance of them developing speech and language skills at a slower pace. Poor literacy skills and difficulty communicating can lead to behavioral problems in your child as they struggle in school (Gordon, 2022).

UNDERSTANDING YOUR BABY'S CUES

Understanding your baby's cues helps with responsive and effective caregiving. There are many common cues that babies use to communicate their needs. You are going to be the expert on your baby almost immediately. You will recognize a tired cry versus a hurt cry before you know it! Trust your parenting gut!

Crying is the primary method that babies express their sorrow or discomfort. It may signify hunger, exhaustion, discomfort, pain, or a demand for attention. Pay attention to the various cries and their cues to better understand your baby's needs.

Signs your baby is hungry include putting their fist to their mouth, sucking on their hands, smacking their lips, opening and closing their mouth, and trying to find your breast or bottle. You should look for these signs when you think your baby is hungry because, by the time they cry, they are already feeling distressed and may have trouble latching or settling into a bottle. Some babies give you ten minutes of non-crying feeding cues, while others give you ten seconds. Let them eat until they are full, when they turn away from the nipple, fall off your breast or bottle, or relax completely and open their fist.

Babies frequently seek eye contact as a means of connecting and communicating. They may look you in the eyes, follow your movements, or make eye contact to convey excitement, recognition, or the desire for reassurance.

Babies express their feelings through facial expressions. They may smile when they are happy, coo and gurgle when they are content, or furrow their brows and frown when upset or uncomfortable. Observing their facial expressions can provide clues to their emotional state.

Babies communicate through their bodies. When they are in pain, they may stiffen their bodies, arch their backs, or pull their legs up to their abdomen if they are experiencing gas or intestinal troubles. When they feel safe and satisfied, they may relax and settle into your arms or your touch.

Babies frequently communicate with their hands and arms. When interested or overstimulated, they may reach for objects, make gripping actions to demonstrate attention, or wave their arms. These movements can reveal information about their interests and preferences.

In addition to crying, newborns make various noises and vocalizations to communicate. They may coo, babble, or produce other sounds to show joy, participate in "conversations," or seek attention. You can reply more appropriately if you pay attention to their vocalizations.

Examine your baby's posture and motions. They may orient their head or body toward a fascinating sound or stimulus, wriggle or wiggle when they want to be put down or moved, or relax and settle when satisfied.

Remember that every baby is unique, and cues vary from one baby to another. Spend time observing and getting to know your baby's cues and patterns. Over time, you will develop a deeper understanding of their needs and preferences, allowing you to respond sensitively and effectively to their cues. Responsive caregiving based on understanding your baby's cues builds trust, strengthens the parent-child bond, and supports your baby's overall development and well-being.

Fostering Communication

When it comes to talking and communicating with babies and toddlers, there are some helpful strategies for interaction, regardless of how young they are. Always ensure they are alert when you talk to them, which helps them stay interested in communication.

Talk to your child a lot. Narrate what you are doing, describe objects, and explain your daily routines. Even if your baby or toddler may not understand all the words, this exposure to language helps develop their vocabulary and language skills. Reading books aloud, even to newborns, can help with vocabulary development. Read the words on the page, but also point to the pictures and describe them or ask questions about what is happening. You can also sing songs or share nursery rhymes. Do this when walking around, driving in the car, getting a bath, or preparing them for bed so they have constant exposure to language.

Be attuned to your child's communication attempts, whether through sounds, gestures, or babbling. Respond promptly and warmly to their attempts to communicate, encouraging them to continue trying to communicate and develop their language skills. If they make eye contact, smile, and reach out to you, this is communication, and you can mirror their actions and respond warmly, smiling and picking them up.

Observe your child's nonverbal cues and body language to understand their needs and emotions. Notice when they show interest, excitement, or frustration, and respond accordingly. This helps your child feel understood and supported. If they point or wave at something, name that item. If they wave at you, wave back to show them the back-and-forth aspect of communication.

Remember, the key is to provide a nurturing and supportive communication environment. By talking, listening, and responding to your child, you create a strong foundation for their language development and overall communication skills from their first months and beyond (Raising Children, 2019).

RESPONSIVE PARENTING

Ask me how many parenting classes I have taken! Parenting is hard work! And while some of it may be intuitive, other aspects may not be. My local school district offered free classes that were very helpful! There are other resources out there as well. Check out the local library, colleges, or universities, or ask your baby's care provider if they have recommendations. These little nuggets of joy do not come out with instructions!

Responsive parenting is a way to respond to your child's needs with warm behaviors, encouraging them to be themselves and showing them that you are attuned to their needs (Edwards, 2014). Seven general principles can help you parent responsively, starting when your baby is a newborn and becoming even more important as they develop into toddlerhood and beyond.

- Show unconditional love
- Have realistic expectations
- Use positive reinforcement instead of punishment
- Connect with your child
- Play with your child
- Help them stay curious
- Celebrate achievements

Show unconditional love. This principle emphasizes the significance of providing your child with unconditional love and support. It involves accepting and valuing your child for who they are, regardless of their actions or accomplishments. Unconditional love contributes to developing a stable attachment between parent and child, promoting emotional well-being and a sense of belonging.

Have realistic expectations. This principle encourages parents to set reasonable and age-appropriate goals for their children. It entails setting expectations considering the child's unique talents, abilities, and developmental stage. Parents can support their child's growth and development while rejecting ego-driven expectations while cultivating their talents and interests.

Use positive reinforcement instead of punishment. Positive reinforcement and rewards are preferred above punishment and discipline in this approach. It involves utilizing encouragement, praise, and rewards to reinforce and motivate your child's desirable behavior. Parents can help children develop self-esteem, confidence, and intrinsic motivation by focusing on positive reinforcement.

Connect with your child. This idea highlights the significance of developing a strong parent-child bond. It involves actively listening, empathizing, and communicating with your child openly and respectfully. Parents may establish trust, promote emotional intelligence, and teach problem-solving skills by prioritizing connection over overreaction to misbehavior.

Play with your child. This principle urges parents to focus on their children's quality time and playfulness. It involves hands-on engagement like pretend play, physical exercises, and face-to-face contact. Parents may focus on creating meaningful and pleasurable experiences by limiting digital distractions, encouraging creativity, and strengthening the parent-child bond.

Help them stay curious. This principle emphasizes the significance of instilling a sense of wonder, curiosity, and a positive attitude in children. It involves promoting discovery, asking questions, and cultivating awe and amazement in the world. Parents may foster resilience, optimism, and a lifetime love of learning by encouraging a positive approach and highlighting the joy of learning.

Celebrate achievements. This principle emphasizes acknowledging and applauding your child's accomplishments and abilities. It entails recognizing their efforts, progress, and skills. At the same time, it discourages a preoccupation with outward affirmation and vanity. Parents can create a healthy self-concept and a growth attitude in their child by stressing competence over beauty or superficial measures of success.

These principles direct parents to foster a loving, supportive, and respectful connection with their baby. They encourage constructive communication, emotional well-being, self-esteem, and overall growth. Responsive parenting entails tailoring these concepts to the individual needs and personalities of both the parent and the kid, thereby creating a caring and empowering environment for growth (Edwards, 2014).

BUILDING A SECURE ATTACHMENT BOND

Secure attachment refers to a healthy and positive emotional bond that develops between a child and their primary caregiver, typically the parent. A strong and secure attachment relationship forms the foundation for the child's social and emotional development.

The child feels safe, secure, and protected in the presence of their caregiver in a secure attachment relationship. They are certain that their requirements for comfort, soothing, and support will be satisfied on a constant basis.

In a stable attachment connection, the caregiver is emotionally present and sensitive to the child's indications and needs. They are aware of the child's signals, offer comfort and reassurance, and address their emotional and physical requirements on a constant basis.

A firmly attached baby feels free to explore their surroundings, knowing that their caregiver is there as a safe haven. They can explore and learn, yet they always return to their caregiver for comfort and support.

Children that are securely attached have open and effective communication with their caregivers. They are at ease expressing their wants, thoughts, and emotions and confident that their caregiver will respond with attention and understanding.

In a stable attachment connection, the caregiver assists the child in regulating their emotions. They provide comfort, soothing, and direction during distress, assisting the child in learning to manage and regulate their emotions successfully.

Secure attachment establishes a solid foundation for resilience. Securely connected children are more likely to develop good coping mechanisms, self-confidence, and a feeling of self-worth. They are more prepared to deal with life's obstacles and stressors (Robinson, 2019).

Benefits of a Secure Attachment Bond

A secure attachment bond between a child and their primary caregiver has numerous benefits for the child's overall development and well-being.

Children with a healthy attachment bond feel emotionally secure and trusting in their relationships. They have confidence in their caregiver's availability and responsiveness to their needs, which promotes a positive self-image and appropriate emotional control.

Securely attached children have greater social skills and build positive interactions with others. They learn how to communicate, empathize, and regulate their emotions through a secure attachment relationship, laying the groundwork for good social interactions.

Secure attachment supports cognitive development. When children feel safe and secure, they are more open to exploring their environment and engaging in learning experiences. They have a strong foundation for curiosity, problem-solving, and positive brain development.

Securely attached children tend to have higher self-esteem and self-confidence. The consistent support and validation they receive from their caregiver help them develop a positive self-image, a belief in their abilities, and a sense of worthiness.

A secure attachment bond provides a safe and supportive environment for children to learn how to regulate their emotions. They develop the ability to recognize and express their feelings appropriately, manage stress, and cope with challenges effectively.

Children with secure attachments are more likely to develop resilience and adaptation. They have a stable foundation from which to explore the world, take risks, and tackle obstacles. Their caregiver's regular support and love help them build coping skills and recover from adversity.

Brain development benefits from secure attachment. Caregiver-child interactions that are caring and responsive increase healthy brain connections, particularly in emotional regulation, social skills, and stress response.

Secure connection lays the groundwork for future good partnerships. Children with a solid attachment link are more likely to create stable and happy relationships later in life with friends, romantic partners, and their children.

Secure attachment is a process that evolves and can be influenced by various factors. However, nurturing a secure attachment bond in the early years of a child's life has long-lasting positive effects on their emotional, social, and cognitive development (Robinson, 2019).

INTERACTIVE ELEMENT

Trying to plan activities to bond with your baby can feel like another task to take on, and, let's be real, easy to procrastinate. So, here is a list of activities you can do to bond with your baby, connect with them, and foster communication.

For babies 0 to 3 months:

- Consider teaching your baby some simple signs so they can communicate with you before they have verbal skills. Many babies can learn the signs for mommy, daddy, book, more, bed, all done, milk, diaper, yes, no, please, and thank you. Learn the signs and use them with your baby to establish communication.
- Narrate what you are doing when you change your baby's diaper or get them dressed. Sing silly rhymes, like "This Little Piggy," while touching their toes to engage with them.
- Talk about who's feeding the baby. If you are breastfeeding or giving your baby a bottle, say, "Mommy is feeding you now." If your partner is

giving the baby a bottle, name your partner; for example, "Daddy is feeding you breakfast."

- After a bath, put lotion on your hands and rub them together to warm them up. Massage it into your baby's skin, naming each part of their body as you touch it.
- Play peek-a-boo with your baby, naming the toy or item in play when you show it to them. Hide it and ask them where it is. Bring it back out and say, "Here it is!"
- Hold your baby close and position them so they can comfortably see your face. Stick out your tongue and keep it there. See if your baby mimics you. Try other facial expressions, like smiling or opening your mouth wide.

Bonus content! Looking ahead, these are fun ways to engage with babies 3 to 6 months:

- Help your baby become more engaged in the changing process. After changing their diaper or getting dressed, hold their hands and count, "One, two, three, up!" and gently pull them into a sitting position. With practice, they will value this routine and be able to sit up more easily.
- When your baby babbles, wait for them to finish, and talk or babble back. This natural give and take will help them understand the flow of conversation.

- When your baby has tummy time, put a mirror in front of their face so they can look at themselves.
- Show your baby pictures of other people, including pictures in your photo albums or books. Identify the emotion on each person's face.
- Take your baby on a nature walk and talk about everything you see and smell. Collect leaves, grass, acorns, sticks, and flowers. When you get home, seal the items into jars so your baby can safely handle them and explore them up close.
- Start reading board books to your baby, letting them grasp the thick pages to help turn them.

KEY TAKEAWAYS

It is easy to get caught up in your healing process and adaptation to motherhood in the postpartum period, but bonding with your baby is so important.

- Bonding can be as simple as skin-to-skin contact, which is especially beneficial right after childbirth. It helps babies adapt to life outside the womb, regulate their temperature, and prepare to feed. It also benefits the mother by helping her bond with the baby, feel love, and produce milk.
- Mindful parenting is an approach that helps you parent your child without letting emotions get in the

way. You will behave mindfully, taking everything in without judgments or reactions.

- Your baby wants to communicate with you even though they do not have verbal skills, much less hand-eye coordination! You can interact with your baby by talking to them, babbling in response to their noises, making eye contact, and even teaching them simple signs.

- Responsive parenting is a way to customize your parenting style to your baby's needs. You connect and play with them, loving them as they are without expectations of who they should be or how they should act.

- A secure attachment style will help your child develop into a confident adult. You can help them feel secure by showing that you are always around to help and support them, reacting sensitively to their needs and comforting them when necessary.

8

PARENTHOOD AND PROGRESS: NAVIGATING WORK, FINANCES, AND GOALS IN POSTPARTUM LIFE

The future depends on what we do in the present.

— MAHATMA GANDHI

After pregnancy, childbirth, and self-care during the fourth trimester, another major transition is coming your way: settling into this new life with routines, whether that involves going back to work, juggling family responsibilities, or being a stay-at-home parent.

TRANSITIONING BACK TO WORK

Maternity leave may be less than you wanted in terms of healing and adapting to your life as a new parent, and you dread juggling work stress with parenting. You might only return because you need the money or fear losing your job. Alternatively, you might be ready to return to work because you love your job and want to start balancing home life with work. However, your feelings about returning to work are valid, so you should not feel guilty.

Even if you are excited to return to work, it can be a tough transition, so you should still prioritize self-care. You do not need to overschedule yourself as you go back to your previous lifestyle. You need to remember that you have a newborn to care for when you get home. You may need to pump during the day if breastfeeding to prevent engorgement and ensure you continue to produce enough milk for your baby.

If you still have paid time off at work, you might want to take a day off every week to catch up with caring for your baby and give yourself some downtime. Whether you have time off or not, you will want to ask for help whenever possible. Just as you delegated things during the fourth trimester, you should consider hiring help, having groceries delivered, and taking people up on their offers of help—whatever ensures you can make time for yourself while juggling work, parenthood, and your partner.

Once you return to work, you can even ask for help from your job. Ask for a private pumping room, which they must provide by law (U.S. Department of Labor, 2020). Meet with your boss and coworkers to get caught up on things that happened while you were out. Some workplaces may offer new moms a flexible schedule, including the chance to work remotely or return part-time for a month before going full-time again. You also need to know that your boss will be flexible with you if your baby gets sick and you need a day off or to work remotely to stay with them.

Talk with your partner about this step because they may be able to change their hours, too. One of you can go to work later to have more time with the baby in the morning, and the other can get off work early to pick the baby up from the caregiver and have time together in the evening.

Starting childcare before you return to work can help you feel more comfortable. You will be available if your baby needs anything, and you will get to know the provider and work out drop-off and pick-up routines. Once you return to work, check in with your caregiver several times during the day. You can get updates about how your baby is doing, which can relieve your anxiety and guilt over going back to work.

As with anything regarding parenting a newborn, there is no right or wrong way to go back to work. You need to do what feels best for you. Take it slow, and do not get overwhelmed, because you are most likely still in a fragile emotional state and do not want to push yourself too far. Ensure your partner, family, and friends support your choices. Ideally, your boss and coworkers will too, but the bottom line is that you have to do what is best for you.

FINANCIAL ASPECTS OF PARENTHOOD

Adapting to life as a parent is a significant change throughout pregnancy, the fourth trimester, and beyond. However, the financial aspects can be just as challenging to manage. There is a reason that so many people never feel prepared to have a baby—you may think that you need to have thousands of dollars stockpiled to get through the first few years, not to mention the growing expense of childcare, healthcare, and education!

Financial stress is a real worry for so many people, but there are ways you can overcome it. Cutting costs and making smart choices when buying supplies for your baby will significantly help you save money while still having everything you need for your little one. While these tips address baby items, you can use many of the same concepts, like buying secondhand and using Facebook Buy Nothing groups, throughout your life, for you and your child.

Financial Stress

It almost seems like a joke that such a tiny new person can be so expensive, but it is a hard truth in life! Depending on your insurance, you may be thousands of dollars in debt due to childbirth bills just as soon as your baby is born. You might also want to pay to have a doula by your side, and that is before you even get into the car seat, stroller, diapers, clothes, ointments, bottles, and endless baby accessories.

Parents report spending anywhere from $7,000 to $14,600 annually for the first two years of their babies' lives (Skolnik, 2023). While you may not be able to keep your financial stress under control, you should try because women who stress about money while pregnant often give birth to babies with lower birth weights (Holland, 2019). You might have lived comfortably as a single person or even with your partner. However, the thought of bringing a baby into your financial situation may make it seem like you do not have enough to provide the necessities.

One of the best ways to reduce stress is to know that your baby does not need much initially. They grow so quickly in the first year that you do not need to spend money on cute outfits they will only wear a couple of times. You will provide them love, attention, and support, which means more than all the outfits and teething rings in the world! If you are truly worried and feel like your anxiety is spiraling, talk to your provider, doula, partner, and support system. Feeling heard and understood, along with getting practical advice, can help alleviate the stress that can have a negative impact on your baby.

You can also take steps to cut costs and leave more money in your pocket. You can still provide everything your baby needs without breaking your budget.

Cutting Costs

If you give birth in a hospital, ask about coupons and free samples. Many brands give maternity wards samples and coupons to help new moms learn what they have to offer. You may get diapers, ointment, lotion, and baby wash. Coupons will help save money on items you need once you are home, so you could ask to see what is available!

Beyond asking, take what you are given! I loved the mesh underwear so much that I packed all the pairs they gave me to take home. When the nurse saw me, she slipped me a few extras! I also took some baby care items with my baby's bassinet, like disposable nipples for bottles and a nasal aspirator. These things were already for my baby, and I know the hospital cannot reuse them, though I asked to make sure!

If you can breastfeed your baby, you will save a lot of money because formula is costly. Not everyone can or wants to nurse, which is fine, but if you are stressed about finances, you might want to try. Formula can cost about $1,400 if you exclusively bottle-feed for the first year, so breastfeeding can save a lot, even if you supplement with formula (Skolnik, 2023). And while it may be free to do, I want to acknowledge that the time and effort into nursing or pumping is priceless!

How can we put a price tag on that? Do not let anyone tell you otherwise!

Many hospitals and parenting resources can help you find free lactation support to help you get the hang of breastfeeding. While you can hire your own lactation consultant, in the vein of saving money, you will want to find free resources. Some breastfeeding organizations help over the phone, via Zoom, or offer home visits if you are local. Doulas can also help you and your baby find the correct latch.

If your baby does not take to the breast, you can use a breast pump to pump milk for bottles instead of formula. If you pump regularly, you will continue to produce milk as if your baby were getting it directly from you. You can borrow a breast pump from a friend since it is expensive. Some health insurance will cover a breast pump for new mothers, so look into that option, too.

You can save money by not buying nursing clothes, too. Nursing bras and tops are incredibly convenient but can cost two or three times more than an average garment. If breastfeeding during your maternity leave, consider wearing loose tops, button-down shirts, or robes during the day so you can easily breastfeed. You can use a baby blanket as a nursing cover instead of buying an expensive, dedicated option.

Next to formula, the most expensive baby item is diapers. Your baby will go through so many diapers in those first three or four years that it will blow your mind! But it does not have to blow your budget! Invest in cloth diapers. You can have two dozen cloth diaper inserts and covers and use them the entire time your baby needs diapers. As you wash diapers, they get softer and more absorbent, so they keep working. Most covers are adjustable, so you can snap them to ensure they fit snugly and comfortably on your baby. Newborn cloth diapers are different, so you may prefer to buy disposable diapers and transition to cloth as your baby grows. You can rinse the diapers in the toilet and then wash them as usual. If they get stained, hang them in the sun to dry and get bleached clean naturally! Once your baby is out of diapers, you can use the inserts as rags or pass them on to a new mom. Cloth diapers are the gift that keeps giving.

Babies are tiny, but they need many *things*. The issue is that they grow and change so quickly that you can feel like you are throwing money away. For example, my friend bought about 20 cute onesies for her newborn. However, since she was doing laundry so much, it turned out that her daughter only wore ten or fewer onesies before she needed to go up to the next size! After that, I learned to give expectant mothers onesies in staggered sizes as a gift. Everyone gives new baby items, but when you reach nine months, you are on your own! Getting bigger sizes of items at baby showers is a great way to know you have the basics covered for your baby's first year, especially since you can launder the onesies and re-wear them often—your baby does not need to be a fashionista just yet!

You can also buy baby clothes at a discount or thrift store. Wash them in your detergent before dressing your baby so you know their skin will not react to what the thrift store uses—if anything! I recommend buying as much plain white stuff as possible, especially for those early months. White onesies, white socks, white bibs. That means you can bleach them in a big batch instead of spot-treating them and having stained or discolored garments. See if any friends or family members have hand-me-down clothes, too, and clean them as you would thrift store garments to keep your baby's skin safe.

Baby shoes are adorable, but you do not need shoes yet. You can pay as much for baby shoes as you do for your own, and they will not even walk in them! Baby shoes also fall off easily, so you might come home with one lost shoe after your first outing. I recommend using socks or, if your baby is born in winter or you live in a cold climate, knit booties that help them retain heat when they are outside. You can also bundle them with layers and a hat to stay warm and tuck a baby blanket around them, so shoes are unnecessary.

If you get gifts you do not want or cannot use, ask a friend who wants to help to return them for you. Baby Gap clothes are cute, but if you do not need them, you can return them for store credit and buy some necessities or get items in a bigger size so you have more for when your baby gets older. If you vow to return items yourself, you might miss the return window because you have a lot of other tasks on your plate at this point.

It is ideal for getting baby items with multiple functions. For example, you can get a changing table that doubles as a dresser—or attach a changing pad to your existing dresser! You can buy cribs that convert to toddler and twin beds as your child grows, only needing to replace the mattress instead of buying something entirely new and disposing of what you had. There are high chairs that convert to booster seats and regular chairs as your baby grows up.

Also, check for compatibility. A car seat is one of the first things you want to get so you are ready whenever the baby comes. But instead of buying a completely random stroller, use your car seat information to find a compatible stroller. That will help you walk with your baby when they are still so young that they need to be in the car seat. You can set it in the stroller and have an easier time on walks or transitioning from the car to a store.

You should pack an extra supply bag to keep in the car—in addition to your regular diaper bag. If your baby spits up or has accidents on your diaper bag items, you have extra diapers, clothes, and ointments in the car. You will not have to stop at the nearest store to buy replacements, which can add up over time.

Finding a lot of fun, free activities for your baby is also possible. While you might love music classes or yoga classes to bond with other new moms, memberships can get pricey. Your library most likely offers free music classes, story times, and other events for babies and parents.

The freebies do not end when you leave the hospital. As you take your baby to regular checkups, ask the pediatrician for samples and coupons. They often have formula and ointment samples they can give you at each appointment. You can sign up for the mailing list of major baby brands and get regular coupons in your email inbox.

Check out the local library! They certainly have books, books, and more books! These can be audiobooks as well. Additionally, there are many other free programs that libraries offer. Art classes, music, movies, exercise groups, and numerous child programs are just a few that our local library offers.

There are other ways to save money with your new baby:

- See if you are eligible for WIC, the federal nutrition program for Women, Infants, and Children.
- Sign up for formula coupons and freebies.
- Buy everything possible used from thrift stores or friends.
- Look for items on Facebook Buy Nothing groups.
- Check for retail sales and coupons you can use on wipes and diapers.
- Invest in cloth diapers to save money in the long run.

- Only buy things as needed since your baby can grow out of them or not need them.
- Put practical items on your baby registry.
- Do not worry about a cute nursery because your baby will sleep in your room for the first six months anyway!
- Join your local library.

When it comes to food after weaning your baby, you can keep costs low, too. You can buy fresh produce and mash it up for your baby when they are ready. While having some baby-friendly snacks on hand can make the feeding process easier, having them eat the same food as the rest of the family makes meal prep more manageable and can help avoid picky eating issues later.

SETTING PERSONAL AND FAMILY GOALS

The focus of the fourth trimester is healing and self-care, but that does not mean you forget all that when it comes to the next phase of life. You can still set personal and family goals to keep your life running smoothly.

Personal goals can include anything that interests you or feels like a priority. You can learn a new hobby or skill for fun or turn it into a business or side hustle. You may want to travel more or volunteer and make a difference in the world. You may prefer to focus on spending time with your family and improving your health and wellness. You may want to pay off debt and become financially independent. There are no right or wrong goals—simply things that matter most to you.

Family goals can also encompass a range of purposes and activities. You may want to feed your family whole foods and meal prep each week in advance, prioritizing dinners together. You could have a family movie night and read together every night as a bedtime routine. You may want to spend more time outside and with friends than in front of electronic screens. You may want to evenly distribute the chores, including age-appropriate tasks, to your children. You can also have bigger goals relating to your house or how you want your life to look. You may want to renovate the house to create an attic playroom for the kids. You can decide to move to a different location to be near a better school district. You can have the goal of paying off debt to travel with your family and homeschool your kids.

You can break big goals down into actionable steps so you can make progress toward them. Continuing the home-schooling example, you can start researching the home-school curriculum while your child is still a baby so you have an idea of the teaching style you can handle and how you would like them to learn. You can start saving money for a big family trip and research how long a visa allows you to stay in a specific country. Start a very small college account that will eventually turn into something great over time. Small steps eventually can turn into large leaps.

Whatever goals you want to make, you should set SMART ones. SMART goals are Specific, Measurable, Achievable, Relevant, and Time-bound. That means you do not just say you want to travel and homeschool your kids in the future. You say you want to travel abroad and live there for six months, homeschooling your children throughout elementary school. To do that, you will need a budget of this much. If you cannot make it happen, have a backup plan. SMART goals can help you achieve what you want in life, whether personal or family, big or small.

INTERACTIVE ELEMENT

Setting SMART goals is a productive way to reach your dreams, but even the thought of finding that purpose can seem overwhelming in the fourth trimester. This worksheet will help you set actionable goals.

	Goal	Why? How?
Smart		
Measurable		
Achievable		
Realistic		
Time-bound		

Here's an example filled in for you.

	Goal	Why? How?
Smart	Make time for self-care	I need time to relax without worrying about the baby.
Measurable	I will factor one hour of self-care into my weeks.	I will ensure I treat it like an appointment, not for fun.
Achievable	I will schedule baby coverage for those hours a month in advance.	My partner or parent can watch the baby for one hour a week.
Realistic	I need to prioritize this time for myself.	I want to stay true to myself and value my mental health.
Time-bound	I will take one hour a week for the next year.	At that time, I can reassess how I feel and what I need for my self-care.

Why? How?

You can use this worksheet for any goal, multiple goals, all the goals! It makes you think about what you want more purposefully, which can improve your chance of actually prioritizing these goals and taking steps to achieve them.

KEY TAKEAWAYS

Making it through the fourth trimester is just the beginning of your motherhood journey! It is important to prioritize your personal and family goals at this point to ensure you are living a full life and following your passions.

- Take it easy when transitioning back to work. Do not hesitate to ask your employer about working part-time, remotely, or flexible hours.

- Start childcare before you go back to work. This lets you get to know the provider and establish a drop-off and pick-up routine with your baby.
- Money can be stressful but do not let it get to you—or your baby. There are many ways to cut costs and live frugally as you adjust to parenthood and caring for your baby physically, emotionally, and financially.
- Think about how you want your life to look. What would you do if you could learn a new hobby, change jobs, travel, or make more time for yourself? Set actionable goals so you can balance yourself with the role of motherhood.
- Talk with your partner about family goals. What do you want to do with your family in the next one, five, or ten years? Make SMART goals to reach your dreams.

9

YOUR POSTPARTUM PLAYBOOK— WINNING THE FIRST 12 WEEKS

IN EVERY CHAOS, THERE IS A COSMOS, IN EVERY DISORDER, A SECRET ORDER. —CARL JUNG

You have learned so much about caring for yourself during the fourth trimester! You know to rest, prioritize nutrition, and accept help from all the supportive people you have around you. As you wrap up this period of your life, you might start to feel like you don't know what comes next.

After getting help and insight from your provider and countless pregnancy books, and now learning so much about the fourth trimester from this book, you might feel like you are about to be left all alone. However, there is no reason to feel that way! Everything you have learned in this book has empowered you to make the right choices in the future. Most importantly, it's helped you understand the importance of trusting yourself. You're a mama now, so you know what is best for yourself and your baby, and you have the tools to implement that lifestyle moving forward.

However, I am not going to leave you hanging. This chapter is all about looking ahead and seeing the bigger picture of parenthood. Instead of getting information you cannot use until your baby is a toddler or school-aged, this stuff will help now.

The planning ahead section gives you ideas of what you need to list on a postpartum plan, just as you mapped out the childbirth process with a birth plan. If you have everything you need in one place, you will feel empowered to make the right choices without needing to take time to stress—or even think, since it's already done for you.

The interactive element helps you even more, with a postpartum planning worksheet you can fill in and use as a jumping-off point. But make sure you include resources that you think you'll need—it's better to have too much information on hand than not enough!

Finally, the week-by-week worksheet helps you understand what might be happening each week after you give birth, but there are also lines where you can fill in your own goals to ensure you stay on the right track and in the right mindset as you experience the fourth trimester and beyond.

EMBRACING POSTPARTUM LIFE LESSONS

It's easy to get caught up in the idea of how life is supposed to be—or how media and social media make you *think* it should be. But there are some honest life lessons that will help you embrace postpartum life.

Most importantly, know that everyone is different. If you have another baby after this, your experience will most likely be different. Your friends who have babies will have different experiences. It's okay that things are different because that means you can be flexible and go with the flow.

That segues right into the life lesson of trusting your instincts. You know your body, and after having your baby, you will have similar feelings about what is best for them. There is nothing wrong with asking for advice from your provider, doula, partner, mom group, or friends, but you will know in your gut if something is right or wrong. Always listen to that because it is most likely correct.

Asking for advice is a great life lesson because it reinforces the idea that no mother is alone. People love to help, so having support for yourself and/or your baby can make a huge difference in your life. It's okay to lean on people some-times because they want to help you, and you can help them in return when they need it. Asking for help is not a weak-ness—it is empowering because you are admitting you cannot do it alone, and people will rise to help you.

That said, you cannot please everyone, so do not even try. There will be people who not only want to give you advice but stand over you to ensure you follow that advice. If it doesn't feel right to you, don't do it, even if it bothers them. You are responsible for yourself and your baby. No one else's feelings matter that much, especially if they are trying to tell you how to be a parent.

Along with your inability to please everyone is the importance of self-care. As I just mentioned, you and your baby are the most important people right now, and you can't take care of your baby if you don't have any energy. You need time to yourself, time to relax, time to recharge. You need to stay in touch with your true self to be the best parent possible. It's not selfish to prioritize yourself sometimes because self-care can make a huge difference in your parenting.

It is also crucial to remember that you do not need to be perfect, and you never will, even if you try. You will just make yourself unhappy and frustrated. It is better to appreciate the small things as they happen, roll with the punches, and grow with each new experience. You will become the best mother you can be, just give yourself the grace and patience to try, fail, and grow. Life is a journey, and this precious time with your baby is something you should appreciate and feel grateful for because it'll be gone in a flash!

PLANNING AHEAD

Many women make a birth plan with their provider, but fewer think ahead to the postpartum plan. You're going to be so exhausted after childbirth that having a road map of what comes next can greatly help you transition into the fourth trimester.

What to Include in Your Postpartum Plan

You have been tracking your body and your baby's progress throughout pregnancy and still monitor things once they're born, so planning should be second nature by now. A postpartum plan can include details such as

- Meal planning resources.
- Options to outsource tasks, like a cleaning company, landscape business, and grocery delivery service.
- A timeline of your maternity leave and when you plan to return to work.
- Childcare options to research.
- Contact information for a doula, lactation consultant, psychologist or counselor, and support group.
- A list of people who can watch the baby when you need a break.
- A schedule showing which partner will take night shifts with the baby.

Include anything in your plan that will help you keep things organized and feel in control when you are home with the baby. Remember that your emotions and hormones may feel all over the place, so having more detailed information can help you feel confident and prepared. It is better to have every little thing written down than not have what you need when you're feeling stressed!

INTERACTIVE ELEMENT

Sample Postpartum Planning Worksheet

For free example copy please go to @imabouttobe OR https://www.instagram.com/imabouttobe/

Parental leave for Mom

_____

and Partner

_____

When Mom returns to work:

_____

When Partner returns to work:

_____

Mother's expected roles:

_____

_____

_____

Partner's expected roles:

_____

_____

_____

What are the night shift hours?

_____

What are the night shift roles/expectations?:

_____

Visitors allowed: #____and names

_____

_____

_____

How visitors can help:

_____

_____

_____

Code word to encourage visitors to leave:

_____

Who can help in the mornings? Name and contact info:

_____

Who can help in the afternoons? Name and contact info:

_____

Who can help at night? Name and contact info:

_____

Frozen meals to prepare:

_____

Grocery stores that deliver:

_____

Restaurants that deliver:

_____

Childcare options to research:

_____

_____

_____

Weekly goals for emotional and physical recovery

Week 1: Adjusting to parenthood

- Take a shower and wash your hair
- Continue peri care or incision care
- Nap as often as possible
- Continue to work on feeding plan
- Schedule follow-up appointment for baby
- Schedule lactation support as needed
- Communicate with partner about new routine

- Get outside and sit in the sun

- _____
- _____
- _____
- _____

Week 2: Building a foundation

- Get more comfortable feeding the baby
- Learn the baby's cues and cries
- Focus on nutrition and meal planning
- Confirm a sleep protection plan for mama to be continued
- Take gentle walks outside
- Journal and process the birth
- Schedule consult with pelvic floor physical therapist as needed
- Follow up with OB care provider as needed
- Start coming out of the initial "birth fog"—if you don't feel this, contact your provider and support team

- _____
- _____
- _____
- _____

Weeks 3–5: Creating routines

- Develop a feeding routine and sleep shifts
- Make a schedule of walks and interactions with your baby
- Delight in your baby focusing on your face
- Have your follow-up baby appointment
- Stitches should dissolve, but continue peri care and incision care as needed

- _____
- _____
- _____
- _____

Weeks 6–9: Get in touch with yourself

- Get a checkup from your provider—physical and mental
- Make sure you're current on your dental exams
- Spend at least two hours a week alone or out of the house
- Establish a weekly "family" meeting to check in with your partner
- See your baby recognize faces
- Notice your baby's communication coos

- _____
- _____
- _____
- _____

Weeks 10–12: Looking to the future

- Plan childcare and your return to work
- Maintain self-care and time with yourself
- Consider what your new routine for physical activity and exercise will look like
- See your baby adjust to tummy time and lift their head
- Track toys with their eyes

- _____
- _____
- _____
- _____

KEY TAKEAWAYS

You're almost there, mama! This chapter was all about helping you look ahead and have a plan in place! How do you feel? Remember:

- Having a postpartum plan is just as helpful as a birth plan. You can have lists of everything you need done while you're in the fourth trimester, and you can use these lists to show people how they can support you!

- Motherhood is a journey. You don't need to be perfect—you will be good enough for your baby if you try! So, let yourself fumble and fail without beating yourself up over it—you'll learn, adapt, and get the hang of this motherhood thing in no time
- Setting small goals or timelines for the first few months after giving birth can help you keep things in perspective. Print the worksheet above and use it so you don't feel overwhelmed or anxious.

If this book was helpful to you, lets spread the word!

Do you know someone that this book could help? Its by your support and reviews that my book is able to reach other pregnant and postpartum families. Please take 60 seconds to kindly leave a review on Amazon. Please scan the QR code below. If you are in a country that isn't listed, please use the link provided by your Amazon order.

Please follow these steps to rate and review my book

- Open your camera on your phone
- Hover over the QR code
- Rate/Review my book

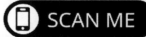

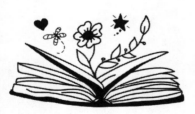

CONCLUSION

Motherhood is an exciting journey that may feel scary or stressful at times, but you should know that you have everything necessary to be an amazing parent already in you! This book's goal was to help you find it. By organizing your life and preparing yourself for your new baby, you can prioritize self-care and healing after childbirth.

So many mothers do not get the postpartum support they need, and it has been my purpose to help you understand how you should treat yourself during the first 12 weeks postpartum. I want to map out the entire experience, so you know what you need to heal and why. I want you to understand the physical changes your body is going through and how to be kind to yourself to allow for healing and acceptance during this time.

By prioritizing your self-care and being open and honest with your partner and support system, I want you to realize that you can be the best mom possible while staying true to yourself. You do not have to let yourself go and become a mom only—there is room for time alone, relaxation, rediscovering your favorite pastimes, and even learning new hobbies. Your world does not get smaller because you had a baby—it grows, because you learn new things about yourself, your little one, your partner, and the family members and friends you thought you already knew. You will see new sides of everyone as they come together in a community for your baby. You will also meet new people who are going through the same phases of life as you.

The worries you have as a new mother are worries that many other moms have had, and I hope I addressed them all in this book. It is easy to feel overwhelmed with your new baby and compare yourself to what you see on social media and in movies, but the best thing you can do at this stage is to be true to yourself. Your baby will love your unique approach to motherhood, even as you navigate the challenges and learn along with your little one. Your heart will continue to grow with each day on this adventure with your baby, so be open to it all.

I hope this book has helped you feel supported during the often-forgotten fourth trimester. If the advice and support in this book helped you, please leave a review so other new mamas know they can find like-minded friends in the pages of this book. Most importantly, go forward in your motherhood journey with an open heart, ready for the excitement of this phase in life!

REFERENCES

A Dime Saved. (2023, May 28). *12 budget-friendly ways to cut costs on baby necessities*. A Dime Saved. https://adimesaved.com/ways-to-cut-costs-on-baby-necessities

Abramson, A. (2022, September 22). *What is weaponized incompetence, and are you guilty of it?* Fatherly. https://www.fatherly.com/life/what-is-weaponized-incompetence

Achwal, A. (2020, October 27). *Is it safe to eat ghee after cesarean delivery?* Parenting.firstcry.com. https://parenting.firstcry.com/articles/is-eating-ghee-after-c-section-delivery-recommended/

Ackerman, C. (2017, October 4). *10+ coping skills worksheets for adults and youth (+ pdfs)*. PositivePsychology.com. https://positivepsychology.com/coping-skills-worksheets/

Adams, L. (2021, April 9). *New mothers: Give yourself a "self-compassion break."* Grow Counseling. https://growcounseling.com/new-mothers-self-compassion/

Alpert, Y. M. (2022, February 1). *Making a postpartum plan: How to prep for parenthood*. The Bump. https://www.thebump.com/a/postpartum-plan

American Academy of Dermatology Association. (n.d.). *Hair loss in new moms*. American Academy of Dermatology Association. https://www.aad.org/public/diseases/hair-loss/insider/new-moms

American Academy of Pediatrics. (2022, June 21). *American academy of pediatrics updates safe sleep recommendations: Back is best*. American Academy of Pediatrics. https://www.aap.org/en/news-room/news-releases/aap/2022/american-academy-of-pediatrics-updates-safe-sleep-recommendations-back-is-best/

Anxiety Canada. (n.d.). *Tool 7: Mindfulness (new moms)*. Anxiety Canada. https://www.anxietycanada.com/articles/tool-7-mindfulness-new-moms/

Baby2Body. (2022, July 29). *Breaking down the top 5 myths about postpartum*. Baby 2 Body. https://www.baby2body.com/blog/breaking-down-the-top-5-myths-about-postpartum

Baker, B., & Yang, I. (2018). Social media as social support in pregnancy and the postpartum. *Sexual & Reproductive Healthcare, 17*(1), 31–34. https://doi.org/10.1016/j.srhc.2018.05.003

Bancoff, A. J. (2018, October 4). *The benefits of having a doula throughout the birthing process.* International Doula Institute. https://internationaldoulainstitute.com/2018/10/the-benefits-of-having-a-doula-throughout-the-birthing-process/?gclid=CjwKCAjwscGjBhAXEiwAswQqNAdjAFhmBGO9k7-B9D_dI4nXe0q8DOB9Y7iLnthQ1TJsGf6AHG-UzxoCDB0QAvD_BwE

Barkin, J. L., & Wisner, K. L. (2013). The role of maternal self-care in new motherhood. *Midwifery, 29*(9), 1050–1055. https://doi.org/10.1016/j.midw.2012.10.001

Bean, C., Hatfield, G., & Lesser, I. (2022, December 15). *Heart rate variability and self-compassion: Two tools to help postpartum mothers make exercise decisions.* The Conversation. https://theconversation.com/heart-rate-variability-and-self-compassion-two-tools-to-help-postpartum-mothers-make-exercise-decisions-193548

Bedaso, A., Adams, J., Peng, W., & Sibbritt, D. (2021). The relationship between social support and mental health problems during pregnancy: A systematic review and meta-analysis. *Reproductive Health, 18*(1). https://doi.org/10.1186/s12978-021-01209-5

Blanton, K. (2022, March 24). *8 scientific benefits of meal prepping.* EverydayHealth.com. https://www.everydayhealth.com/diet-nutrition/scientific-benefits-of-meal-prepping/

BlueCross BlueShield. (2020, June 17). *Trends in pregnancy and childbirth complications in the U.S.* BCBS. https://www.bcbs.com/the-health-of-america/reports/trends-in-pregnancy-and-childbirth-complications-in-the-us

Booth, S. (2021, July 25). *Nutrition you need after childbirth.* WebMD. https://www.webmd.com/parenting/baby/nutrition-guide-new-moms

California Department of Health Care Services. (n.d.). *Doula services.* DHCS. https://www.dhcs.ca.gov/provgovpart/Pages/Doula-Services.aspx

Carl Jung Depth Psychology. (2020, July 23). *Carl Jung quote.* Carl Jung Depth Psychology. https://carljungdepthpsychologysite.blog/2020/07/23/carl-jung-in-all-chaos-there-is-a-cosmos-in-all-disorder-a-secret-order/#.ZGJyQHbMKUk

Ceder, J. (2017, October 6). *Mindful parenting: How to respond instead of react.*

The Gottman Institute. https://www.gottman.com/blog/mindful-parent ing-how-to-respond-instead-of-react/

Chamlou, N. (2023, January 3). *Best nutrients for postpartum recovery.* Forbes Health. https://www.forbes.com/health/family/best-postpar tum-recovery/

Chavda, J. (2023, April 13). *In a growing share of U.S. marriages, husbands and wives earn about the same.* Pew Research Center's Social & Demographic Trends Project. https://www.pewresearch.org/social-trends/2023/04/13/ in-a-growing-share-of-u-s-marriages-husbands-and-wives-earn-about- the-same/

Cherry, K. (2023, March 11). *The big five personality traits.* Verywell Mind. https://www.verywellmind.com/the-big-five-personality-dimensions- 2795422

Cleveland Clinic. (n.d.). *Breast engorgement: Causes, complications & treatment.* Cleveland Clinic. https://my.clevelandclinic.org/health/symptoms/ 24306-breast-engorgement

Cleveland Clinic. (2017, January 26). *Bonding with your new baby? 4 kangaroo care benefits.* Health Essentials from Cleveland Clinic. https://health.cleve landclinic.org/4-top-benefits-skin-to-skin-contact-for-babies/

Cleveland Clinic. (2018). *Physical changes after child birth.* Cleveland Clinic. https://my.clevelandclinic.org/health/articles/9682-pregnancy-physical- changes-after-delivery

Cleveland Clinic. (2019). *Omega-3 fatty acids.* Cleveland Clinic. https://my. clevelandclinic.org/health/articles/17290-omega-3-fatty-acids

Cleveland Clinic. (2022a, April 12). *Postpartum depression: Types, symptoms, treatment & prevention.* Cleveland Clinic. https://my.clevelandclinic.org/ health/diseases/9312-postpartum-depression

Cleveland Clinic. (2022b, September 13). *Postpartum psychosis: What it is, symp- toms & treatment.* Cleveland Clinic. https://my.clevelandclinic.org/health/ diseases/24152-postpartum-psychosis

Crouch, M. (2022, July 5). *6 myths about postpartum recovery, from a physical therapist.* Healthline. https://www.healthline.com/health/fitness/postpar tum-recovery-myths

Davis, E. (2023, January 25). *Postpartum hormones: What to really expect after birth.* Endocrine Web. https://www.endocrineweb.com/pregnancy/post partum-hormones

Davis, T. (n.d.). *Personality traits: 430 traits, definition, lists, & examples.* The Berkeley Well-Being Institute. https://www.berkeleywellbeing.com/personality-traits.html

De Sousa Machado, T., Chur-Hansen, A., & Due, C. (2020). First-time mothers' perceptions of social support: Recommendations for best practice. *Health Psychology Open, 7*(1), 205510291989861. https://doi.org/10.1177/2055102919898611

Dennis, C.-L., Fung, K., Grigoriadis, S., Robinson, G. E., Romans, S., & Ross, L. (2007). *Traditional postpartum practices and rituals: a qualitative systematic review.* The Embryo Project Encyclopedia. https://embryo.asu.edu/pages/traditional-postpartum-practices-and-rituals-qualitative-systematic-review-2007-cindy-lee

Diener, E., Lucas, R. E., & Cummings, J. A. (2019, June 28). *Personality traits.* Openpress.usask.ca; University of Saskatchewan Open Press. https://openpress.usask.ca/introductiontopsychology/chapter/personality-traits/

DiMaggio, E. (n.d.). *Promoting self-care for new mothers.* JCFS. https://www.jcfs.org/blog/promoting-self-care-new-mothers

Edwards, B. G. (2014, July 15). *7 principles for responsive parenting.* GoodTherapy.org Therapy Blog. https://www.goodtherapy.org/blog/7-principles-for-responsive-parenting-0715144

Enriquez, T. (2019, April 29). *10 postpartum body affirmations.* Trisha Enriquez. https://trishaenriquez.com/blog/10postpartumbodyaffirmations

Fisher, W. (n.d.). *4 steps to build a unified front as parents.* Dr. Wyatt Fisher. https://www.drwyattfisher.com/blogs/marriage-blog/sharing-power-as-parents

Fletcher, J. (2016, May 17). *4 tips to connect with your partner after having a baby.* Psych Central. https://psychcentral.com/relationships/tips-to-help-reconnect-with-your-partner-after-baby

Fulghum Bruce, D. (2003, March 25). *Postpartum depression.* WebMD. https://www.webmd.com/depression/guide/postpartum-depression

Goodreads. (n.d.-a). *A quote by L.R. Knost.* Goodreads. https://www.goodreads.com/quotes/8418548-taking-care-of-yourself-doesn-t-mean-me-first-it-means

Goodreads. (n.d.-b). *A quote by Mahatma Gandhi.* Goodreads. https://www.goodreads.com/quotes/806111-the-future-depends-on-what-we-do-in-the-present

Gordon, S. (2022, November 21). *Storytime: Why you should be reading to your baby*. Verywell Family. https://www.verywellfamily.com/why-reading-to-babies-is-important-5189827

Griffin, R. M. (2008, April 16). *Magnesium*. WebMD. https://www.webmd.com/diet/supplement-guide-magnesium

Groves, O. (2022, April 7). *25 postpartum journaling prompts for new moms*. Silk + Sonder. https://www.silkandsonder.com/blogs/news/25-journaling-prompts-for-new-moms

Hatfield, J. (2016, August 12). *Dealing with postpartum sleep deprivation*. Postpartum Progress. https://postpartumprogress.com/dealing-postpartum-sleep-deprivation

Henton, S., & Swanson, V. (2023). A mixed-methods analysis of the role of online social support to promote psychological wellbeing in new mothers. *DIGITAL HEALTH, 9*, 205520762211474. https://doi.org/10.1177/20552076221147433

Hill, P. D., Aldag, J. C., Chatterton, R. T., & Zinaman, M. (2005). Psychological distress and milk volume in lactating mothers. *Western Journal of Nursing Research, 27*(6), 676–693. https://doi.org/10.1177/0193945905277154

Holland, K. (2019, April 5). *Pregnancy and financial stress*. Healthline. https://www.healthline.com/health-news/financial-stress-can-affect-unborn-child

Hoyert, D. (2023, March 16). *Maternal mortality rates in the United states, 2021*. CDC. https://www.cdc.gov/nchs/data/hestat/maternal-mortality/2021/maternal-mortality-rates-2021.htm

Hunt, L. (n.d.). *#HealthQuote*. Pinterest. Retrieved May 15, 2023, from https://www.pinterest.ph/pin/healthquote-the-groundwork-of-all-happiness-is-good-health--359091770262792168/

Jiang, L., & Zhu, Z. (2022). Maternal mental health and social support from online communities during pregnancy. *Health & Social Care in the Community, 30*(6). https://doi.org/10.1111/hsc.14075

Johnson, T. C. (2023, April 19). *What to do if you have postpartum hemorrhoids*. WebMD. https://www.webmd.com/baby/what-to-do-if-you-have-postpartum-hemorrhoids

Johnston, Y. (2021, June 2). *The effects of postpartum sleep deprivation*. Hello Postpartum™. https://hellopostpartum.com/postpartum-sleep-deprivation/

Lambermon, F., Vandenbussche, F., Dedding, C., & van Duijnhoven, N. (2020). Maternal self-care in the early postpartum period: An integrative review. *Midwifery, 90,* 102799. https://doi.org/10.1016/j.midw.2020. 102799

Lambert, L. (2020, October 4). *Pregnancy, parenting, lifestyle, beauty: Tips & advice.* Mom.com. https://mom.com/baby/a-few-key-4th-trimester-mile stones-week-by-week/the-4th-trimester-for-moms

Leistikow, N. (2022, December 13). Sleep can help new moms avoid depression. Partners need to do more. *Washington Post.* https://www.washington post.com/wellness/2022/12/09/pregnancy-depression-postpartum-sleep/

Lewis, R. (2020, September 29). *The mother wound: What it is and how to heal.* Healthline. https://www.healthline.com/health/mother-wound

Lindberg, S. (2020a, January 27). *8 postnatal exercises, plus a sample workout you'll love.* Healthline. https://www.healthline.com/health/exercise-fitness/postnatal-exercises

Lindberg, S. (2020b, July 31). *Postpartum diet plan: Tips for healthy eating after giving birth.* Healthline. https://www.healthline.com/health/postpartum-diet

Logan, J. A. R., Justice, L. M., Yumuş, M., & Chaparro-Moreno, L. J. (2019). When children are not read to at home. *Journal of Developmental & Behavioral Pediatrics, 40*(5), 383–386. https://doi.org/10.1097/dbp. 0000000000000657

Major, M. (2020, March 26). *What postpartum care looks like worldwide, and how the U.S. compares.* Healthline. https://www.healthline.com/health/preg nancy/what-post-childbirth-care-looks-like-around-the-world-and-why-the-u-s-is-missing-the-mark

March of Dimes. (n.d.). *Policy and advocacy topics.* March of Dimes.https:// www.marchofdimes.org/policy-and-advocacy-topics

Matrescence Skin. (2023, February 24). *Love your lines: Embracing your body as a mom.* Matrescence Skin. https://www.matrescenceskin.com/blogs/moth erhood-refined/love-your-lines

Mayo Clinic. (n.d.-a). *Sex after pregnancy: Set your own timeline.* Mayo Clinic. https://www.mayoclinic.org/healthy-lifestyle/labor-and-delivery/in-depth/sex-after-pregnancy/art-20045669

Mayo Clinic. (n.d.-b). *Vaginal tears in childbirth.* Mayo Clinic. https://www.

mayoclinic.org/healthy-lifestyle/labor-and-delivery/in-depth/vaginal-tears/art-20546855

Mayo Clinic. (2017). *Relaxation techniques: Try these steps to reduce stress.* Mayo Clinic. https://www.mayoclinic.org/healthy-lifestyle/stress-management/in-depth/relaxation-technique/art-20045368

Mayo Clinic. (2018a). *Postpartum depression - diagnosis and treatment.* Mayo Clinic https://www.mayoclinic.org/diseases-conditions/postpartum-depression/diagnosis-treatment/drc-20376623

Mayo Clinic. (2018b, September 1). *Postpartum depression - symptoms and causes.* Mayo Clinic. https://www.mayoclinic.org/diseases-conditions/postpartum-depression/symptoms-causes/syc-20376617

MGH Center for Women's Mental Health. (2015, July 22). *Postpartum depression: Who is at risk?* MGH Center for Women's Mental Health. https://womensmentalhealth.org/posts/postpartum-depression-who-is-at-risk/

Mikulak, A., & Wolpert, S. (2013, March 4). *Pregnant mothers with strong family support less likely to have postpartum depression.* UCLA. https://newsroom.ucla.edu/releases/stress-hormone-foreshadows-postpartum-243844

Mishra, S. (2022, September 26). *Postpartum fatigue: Know the symptom, cause & remedies.* Freshly Moms. https://www.freshlymoms.com/blogs/news/postpartum-tiredness-or-adrenal-fatigue

Mom in the Six. (2019, July 16). *94 quotes about being a mom in every season of motherhood—mom in the six.* Mom in the Six. https://mominthesix.com/quotes-about-being-mom/

Motroni, A. (2023, May 1). *DIY postpartum padsicles.* The Postpartum Party. https://thepostpartumparty.com/easy-diy-padsicles/

Negron, R., Martin, A., Almog, M., Balbierz, A., & Howell, E. A. (2013). Social support during the postpartum period: Mothers' views on needs, expectations, and mobilization of support. *Maternal and Child Health Journal, 17*(4), 616–623. https://doi.org/10.1007/s10995-012-1037-4

Olson, A. (2020, September 6). *10 ways to improve sleep during pregnancy and postpartum.* Kyte Baby. https://kytebaby.com/blogs/news/10-ways-to-improve-sleep-during-pregnancy-and-postpartum

Osuman, S. (2022, September 7). *Postpartum body quotes—motivation and love.* Motivation and Love. https://motivationandlove.com/postpartum-body-quotes?utm_content=bd-true

Pacheco, D., & Vyas, N. (2020, December 18). *Sleep deprivation and postpartum depression.* Sleep Foundation. https://www.sleepfoundation.org/preg nancy/sleep-deprivation-and-postpartum-depression

Pallarito, K. (2021, August 27). *Your postpartum nutrition guide.* What to Expect. https://www.whattoexpect.com/first-year/postpartum/postpartum-diet-nutrition-questions-answered/

Peterson, T. J. (2020, September 24). *Mindful parenting: How it works, benefits, and how to practice.* Choosing Therapy. https://www.choosingtherapy.com/mindful-parenting/

Phillips, H. (2022, April 8). *What causes postpartum insomnia? And how to get rest.* Verywell Family. https://www.verywellfamily.com/what-causes-postpar tum-insomnia-5216136

Philpott, B. (n.d.). *5 ways to connect with your partner after having a baby.* Kindred Bravely. https://www.kindredbravely.com/blogs/bravely/how-to-connect-with-your-partner

Psych Central. (2021, September 28). *One-Minute mindfulness exercises.* Psych Central. https://psychcentral.com/health/minute-mindfulness-exercis es#1-minute-exercises

Raising Children. (2019, November 19). *Talking with babies and toddlers: How to do it and why.* Raising Children Network. https://raisingchildren.net.au/babies/connecting-communicating/communicating/talking-with-babies-toddlers

Robinson, L. (2019). *Building a secure attachment bond with your baby.* HelpGuide.org. https://www.helpguide.org/articles/parenting-family/building-a-secure-attachment-bond-with-your-baby.htm

Root & Rise. (2020, December 1). *Postpartum care must-have items.* Root & Rise. https://www.rootandriseblog.com/the-postpartum-care-must-have-items/

Ruiz, B. (2021, January 16). *How to love and accept yourself as a new mom.* Hello Postpartum™. https://hellopostpartum.com/love-your-self-new-mom/

Schiedel, B. (2023, February 9). *17 mind-blowing ways your body changes after giving birth.* Todays Parent. https://www.todaysparent.com/baby/postpar tum-care/mind-blowing-ways-your-body-changes-after-giving-birth/

Schneider, H. (2022, September 25). *Too many people don't know about post-partum doulas, and that needs to change.* Well+Good. https://www.welland good.com/postpartum-doula-duties-role/

Seitz, J. (2017, July 18). *The importance of skin-to-skin with baby after delivery.*

Sanford Health News. https://news.sanfordhealth.org/childrens/the-importance-of-skin-to-skin-after-delivery-you-should-know/

Simen, G. (2022, June 23). *How to transition back to work after maternity leave.* Hello Postpartum^{TM}. *https://hellopostpartum.com/transition-back-to-work-after*-maternity-leave

Skolnik, D. (2023, May 31). *26 ways to save money when you have a newborn.* Parents. https://www.parents.com/parenting/money/family-finances/32-ways-to-save-money-when-you-have-a-baby/

Stines, Y. (2023, March 1). *Why you need vitamin D3.* Verywell Health. https://www.verywellhealth.com/vitamin-d3-5082500

Suttie, J. (2016, June 13). *How mindful parenting differs from just being mindful.* Mindful. https://www.mindful.org/mindful-parenting-may-keep-kids-trouble/

Taylor, B. (2021, June 10). *Mums Alone: Exploring the Role of Isolation and Loneliness in the Narratives of Women Diagnosed with Perinatal Depression.* Journal of Clinical Medicine. https://www.ncbi.nlm.nih.gov/pmc/arti cles/PMC8197355

Terreri, C. (2018, August 15). *When is it safe to take baby out in public?* Lamaze International. https://www.lamaze.org/Giving-Birth-with-Confidence/GBWC-Post/when-is-it-safe-to-take-baby-out-in-public

The Commonwealth Fund. (2020, February 6). *Measuring maternal mortality.* Common Wealth Fund. https://www.commonwealthfund.org/blog/2020/measuring-mater nal-mortality

The Healthy Mommy. (2019, August 9). *Study finds being pregnant is the same as running a 40-week marathon!* The Healthy Mommy US. https://www.thehealthymommy.com/pregnant-physical-intensity-athletes/

The Motherhood Center of New York. (2022, June 29). *What are perinatal mood and anxiety disorders (pmads)?* The Motherhood Center of New York. https://themotherhoodcenter.com/blog/2022/06/29/what-are-perinatal-mood-and-anxiety-disorders-pmads/

Tiny Buddha. (n.d.-a). *Dan Millman quote.* Tiny Buddha. https://tinybuddha. com/wisdom-quotes/you-dont-have-to-control-your-thoughts-you-just-have-to-stop-letting-them-control-you/

Tiny Buddha. (n.d.-b). *Leo F. Buscaglia quote.* Tiny Buddha. Retrieved May 15, 2023, from https://tinybuddha.com/wisdom-quotes/a-loving-relation

ship-is-one-in-which-the-loved-one-is-free-to-be-himself-to-laugh-with-me-but-never-at-me-to-cry-with-me-but-never-because-of-me-to-love-life-to-love-himself-to-love-b/

U.S. Department of Labor. (2020). *Frequently asked questions – break time for nursing mothers.* Dol.gov. https://www.dol.gov/agencies/whd/nursing-mothers/faq

Unicef. (2023). *Skin-to-skin contact.* Baby Friendly Initiative; UNICEF. https://www.unicef.org.uk/babyfriendly/baby-friendly-resources/implementing-standards-resources/skin-to-skin-contact/

UPMC Magee-Womens Hospital. (2019, November 13). *The importance of a support system for new parents.* UPMC HealthBeat. https://share.upmc.com/2019/11/newborn-support-system/

Vinopal, L. (2022, August 1). *If you're a dad who didn't immediately love your newborn, blame biology.* Fatherly. https://www.fatherly.com/health/why-dads-dont-instantly-bond-with-babies

White, J. (2022, October 19). *How much water should breastfeeding moms drink?* Verywell Family. https://www.verywellfamily.com/does-drinking-more-water-affect-breastfeeding-284285

WIC Breastfeeding. (n.d.). *Baby's hunger cues.* Wicbreastfeeding.fns.usda.gov. https://wicbreastfeeding.fns.usda.gov/babys-hunger-cues

Made in the USA
Las Vegas, NV
02 June 2024

90640324R00127